YOUR PERSONAL REVOLUTION

PRAISE FOR THE BOOK

'A valuable resource for anyone looking to achieve a life transformation, everything you need to succeed has been covered. This book is a great read and challenged my thinking around my own health and fitness routines.'

DANIEL HILL, REGIONAL SALES MANAGER, LINKEDIN, SYDNEY AUSTRALIA

'Implementing the five steps laid out in this book was a game changer for me, highly recommend it if you're wanting to take your health and fitness to the next level.'

DANIEL OTT, PRESIDENT, TRUE NORTH TINY HOMES INC. TORONTO CANADA

'If you've always struggled to keep a consistent health and fitness routine, reading Your Personal Revolution will give you the tools you need to finally feel like you're in control again!'

ADAM RIZWANI, PRESIDENT & MANAGING DIRECTOR STLTH VAPE TORONTO CANADA

'I've always struggled with my weight and motivation to workout. For the first time ever I've been able to commit to a consistent routine thanks to the easy step by step process in this book. Wish I had come across it sooner!'

PATRICK FARRELL, FOUNDER, CLARITY POOL MANAGEMENT, SYDNEY AUSTRALIA

'Jay's is one of the most inspiring leaders in his industry...he doesn't just motivate you, he has you think like an athlete and coaches you to pull out your best.'

LINDA LAURIDSEN, OWNER, THE STYLE SHERPA TORONTO CANADA

Your Personal Revolution: Five Steps to Taking Back Control of Your Health & Fitness
Copyright © 2021 by Jay Quarmby.
All rights reserved.

Published by Grammar Factory Publishing, an imprint of MacMillan Company Limited.

No part of this book may be used or reproduced in any manner whatsoever without the prior written permission of the author, except in the case of brief passages quoted in a book review or article. All enquiries should be made to the author.

Grammar Factory Publishing
MacMillan Company Limited
25 Telegram Mews, 39th Floor, Suite 3906
Toronto, Ontario, Canada
M5V 3Z1

www.grammarfactory.com

Quarmby, Jay, 1983–
Your Personal Revolution: Five Steps to Taking Back Control of Your Health & Fitness / Jay Quarmby

Paperback ISBN 978-1-989737-27-9
eBook ISBN 978-1-989737-28-6

1. HEA007000 Health & Fitness / Exercise / General. 2. HEA038000 Health & Fitness / Work-Related Health. 3. HEA019000 Health & Fitness / Diet & Nutrition / Weight Loss.

Production Credits
Printed in Canada
Cover design by Designerbility
Interior layout design by Dania Zafar
Book production and editorial services by Grammar Factory Publishing

Grammar Factory's Carbon Neutral Publishing Commitment
From January 1st, 2020 onwards, Grammar Factory Publishing is proud to be neutralizing the carbon footprint of all printed copies of its authors' books printed by or ordered directly through Grammar Factory or its affiliated companies through the purchase of Gold Standard-Certified International Offsets.

Disclaimer
The material in this publication is of the nature of general comment only and does not represent professional advice. It is not intended to provide specific guidance for particular circumstances, and it should not be relied on as the basis for any decision to take action or not take action on any matter which it covers. Readers should obtain professional advice where appropriate, before making any such decision. To the maximum extent permitted by law, the author and publisher disclaim all responsibility and liability to any person, arising directly or indirectly from any person taking or not taking action based on the information in this publication.

YOUR PERSONAL REVOLUTION

Five Steps to Taking Back Control of Your Health & Fitness

JAY QUARMBY

To my hottie pottie Lucy, I've experienced many Personal Revolutions throughout my life, but the most significant and most transformative, was the day I met you.

CONTENTS

Introduction: It's Time to Take Back Control	1
Chapter 1: Five Rules to Win Your Personal Revolution	13
Chapter 2: Clarity, Part 1	30
Chapter 3: Clarity, Part 2	49
Chapter 4: Measure	62
Chapter 5: Discipline	77
Chapter 6: Nutrition	96
Chapter 7: Exercise	123
Conclusion: Your Life, Your Potential, Your Revolution	145
A Small Request	154
Acknowledgements	155
About the Author	158

INTRODUCTION

IT'S TIME TO TAKE BACK CONTROL

I'm sick of feeling tired.
I'm sick of being overweight.
I'm sick of having low self-esteem.
I'm sick of feeling weak and afraid to try anything different or physical because I don't know if I can do it.
I'm sick of sitting on the dock while others swim because I hate how I look in swimmers.

Does any of this resonate with you?

If the answer is yes, it's time to embark on a Personal Revolution.

What is a Personal Revolution?

In order to answer that question, let's look at the word 'revolution'. A revolution, by definition, is:

- 'A forcible overthrow of a government or social order, in favour of a new system', or
- 'A drastic political or social change that usually occurs relatively quickly.'

When it comes to a Personal Revolution, it's the same idea. You need to overthrow the 'government' that is running your daily routine, your choices and your habits – specifically in relation to your health and fitness. In short, you need a new system!

When you think of revolutions throughout history, they generally happen because citizens are so unhappy that they reach a breaking point, rise up and make a change. This concept also applies to you in your daily life. You get to a point where you've simply had enough and need to change NOW!

For many people, the focus then shifts to 'taking control' of their life. But what does that really mean? And is it being done in the right way?

WHEN 'TAKING CONTROL' DOESN'T WORK

These days, people try to take control of their lives in all sorts of different ways. It's important to briefly touch on some of these, and why they don't work long term, so that you can identify if some of these relate to you. That way, you can start to see where you are going wrong, and why maybe you haven't been maintaining the healthy lifestyle that you've been wanting.

The most common way people try to take control of their life is by focusing on their career. The more their personal lives fall apart around them, the more they just put their head down and work. Working hard creates a nice blanket of distraction, and a ready supply of excuses for why they aren't working out, why they aren't eating well, why they aren't taking care of themselves, and so on.

As you become more successful, your career starts to define who you are, and your peers start to validate you as a 'successful' person. This strokes your ego, making it easier to ignore the fact that, when you come home and look in the mirror, you hate what you see. Worse than that, though, is the fact that you're always tired, stressed and overworked, with no time for anything outside of work.

Another common way people try to take control of their life is by attempting to change everything negative at once. They get to the point of being fed up with their situation, so they join the nearest gym, hire a trainer, start eating salads for lunch, and start to feel good. However, without any actual game plan, they end up giving up and, all too soon, are back where they started.

I really feel sorry for these people because they are at least trying to make their life better. They have the right intention and recognize that things need to change. But without understanding and following the right sequence, the changes only last a few months, if that. It becomes a never-ending loop of *almost* living the life they want, but eventually falling off the wagon, and taking months, if not years, to attempt to get back on. If this is your experience, this book is written for you, because you are ready to make a change, you sort of know what to do (but not really), and this time you want to do it right.

DO YOU REALLY NEED A PERSONAL REVOLUTION?

Now that you understand what a Personal Revolution is, you may be skeptical as to whether you really need one. Perhaps you're taking control of your life, bit by bit, and are reasonably happy with your progress – even if you're not entirely sure what your ultimate goal is.

Let me ask you this: Which revolutions throughout history were successful? Ones where the people just grabbed a gun or pitchfork and stormed the city hall? Or the ones with strategy plans put in place, the ones with an organized effort – a game plan? I think the answer is obvious.

As tempting as it is to just suddenly start eating better, working out regularly, going to bed earlier, trying to do some yoga, trying to meal prep, trying to lose weight, trying not to eat sugar, and so on, this approach isn't going to work. If you go back to the revolution analogy, the government (your habits, and your normal way of living) is just going to pull out the big guns and destroy you before you have truly taken control!

You need a revolution to occur, so that you can bring down the walls and gates you've built up around yourself to allow the new and improved version of you to emerge. The first thing the revolution fighters do, when they've taken over, is put a chain around the statue of their dictator and rip it down, replacing it with a statue of their new leader. What a great image – tearing down your old self and installing a new leader.

So, as you and I go through this book together, I'll be showing you how to formulate your own secret battle plans, and how to tear down those gates and walls, so you can rise up and overthrow those bad habits and negative behaviours that govern your life.

You may think you're alone in this, but *everyone* needs a Personal Revolution, multiple times throughout their lives. Perhaps you can even recall an instance where you've had one – a time when you reached a breaking point, you created a plan to change your situation, you executed it, and you changed your life. For sure you can think of times when you've at least attempted one. Just think back to any January 1st of any year, if you've been inspired by a New Year's Resolution. Every gym around the world is filled with people trying to take back control of their neglected health and fitness.

If you aren't truly happy with the way you are living your life, if you aren't as healthy and as fit as you want to be, if you look in the mirror and don't have the self-confidence and love for yourself that you should have, then you need a Personal Revolution.

Let me share Doctor Mike Daley's story with you. He needed a Personal Revolution and he contacted me to help him achieve one. Together, we worked through my five-step method (more on this soon) and the results were transformative. Here's what Mike had to say...

MIKE'S STORY

'On my fiftieth birthday, I was thirty pounds overweight and suffering from increasingly frequent bouts of lower back spasms. The weight, I had got used to – I had accepted it as my body type. But the back spasms were more worrisome. I could injure myself by carrying a heavy bag of groceries the wrong way, and it would result in agonizing pain and stiffness. Only lying down flat or standing alleviated the pain, which would last for a few days every time it happened. I travel a lot for work, and I dreaded the idea of folding into an airplane seat for a few hours. It was really beginning to affect my life quality and productivity, which, for someone who runs their own business, is especially worrisome.

'I had spent my entire adult life avoiding exercise, other than walking, and was eating and drinking too much. Sometimes I thought about doing something about it, but I didn't know how to start. I started going to Iyengar yoga classes with my wife and, as difficult as it was, I began to make progress. The back spasms kept happening though. Another guy in the yoga class suggested that I should find a trainer to help me build up core strength. It hadn't occurred to me that my lack of fitness was contributing to the injuries. That's when I found Jay.

'One of the first things he did with me was to sit me down and we really unpacked all the reasons why I hadn't dedicated any time to my fitness and why now it was so important to me to start this new journey. Until now I had never taken the time to really understand why fitness was important to me. I always assumed, as an academic, that fitness and wellness weren't what I needed to focus on – I would leave that to the gym jocks.

'We then did a deep dive into my eating and nutritional habits. This was instrumental in me losing the extra weight I had gained over the years and allowed me to be much more purposeful about how much and what I now eat. For the first time, I really understood the impact my diet choices were having on my life. I haven't had back pain in years now, and when my wife and I go on holidays we aren't limited by my fitness level. For the first time ever, I've found her asking me to slow down on a long flight of stairs, instead of patiently waiting for me to get to the top.'

MY OWN PERSONAL REVOLUTION

My name is Jay Quarmby. I was raised in the Land Down Under, in Sydney, Australia. At the age of twenty-five, I packed my bags and – with a small handful of money, a lot of courage and determination, and some luck – I moved to Toronto, Canada.

Throughout my life, I have needed a Personal Revolution more times than I can remember, but I will share with you what I think is the first time I experienced one, which changed the path I took for the rest of my life.

When I was seventeen, I was searching for social acceptance at a time in life when dating, popularity and confidence seemed completely out of reach. I had never had a girlfriend, and never got picked first for any sports team. I had a small group of friends but, apart from that, I was pretty insignificant to anyone else around me. I was in my last year of high school, and I was completely lost in terms of what I wanted to do with my life.

One day I signed up to my local gym and gingerly walked over to the closest machine. I had no idea what I was doing there. Across from me was a guy, 100 pounds heavier, jacked and intimidating. He sensed my insecurities and said, *'Bro, you're looking to get big, aren't you? You need to start eating kebabs – lots of kebabs.'* For the first time in my life, I felt accepted, in a place where the personal journey becomes the gift, not the results you're hoping to achieve.

From that day on, I kept working out. I started studying fitness and nutrition, and reading every bodybuilding and fitness magazine out there. I started learning about supplements, too. I would spend hours at the local supplement store, talking to the owner about each product, asking him what they did, why you would take them, and so on. As I started to see the results of positive changes, both physically and mentally, my confidence grew and other people around me began to notice.

Within a year, I had friends asking to work out with me, so I had become a personal trainer without even realizing it. That Personal Revolution transformed my entire life and led me all the way from Australia to Canada, where I've helped thousands of people transform their own lives through my one-on-one coaching services, small group workshops, and boot camp program.

Before starting my first personal training business, Southern Cross Fitness, in 2010, I worked for a gym in the downtown core of Toronto, working my way up the ladder from personal trainer to head trainer, group fitness manager and finally functional training director. I now own a company called Personal Revolution – Fitness and Lifestyle Coaching. I work with top-tier executives whose health and personal lives have been neglected due to their careers. I specialize in stepping in at the point of breakdown to help them embark on a Personal Revolution.

One of my biggest advantages and a key reason for my success is that by receiving my education in the highly regulated, leading fitness industry in the world, Australia, I've been uniquely set apart from my competition. Unfortunately, the fitness industry here in Canada is poorly regulated and without a standardized, nationwide educational system.

My boot camp was recognized as one of the top fitness programs in Toronto two years running. In 2016, I was named top trainer in Eastern Canada by *IMPACT Magazine*. I'm regularly called upon to give advice and beta test new fitness products. Most recently, I was the trainer voice for a new running app in development. More than fifty per cent of my clients have worked with me for ten-plus years and I work almost exclusively on a referral basis.

One fun little fact about me: In 2012, I briefly represented Canada in a rugby league tournament in the United States. My international rugby league career was very short lived, and not as impressive as it sounds, but it's a claim to fame that I enjoy touting every now and then.

So, why did I write this book – and how can it help you?

A FIVE-STEP PROCESS TO YOUR PERSONAL REVOLUTION

I wrote this book for one simple reason: I wanted to give you an opportunity to experience your own Personal Revolution. I honestly believe that if someone can improve their life, feel good about themselves and start to love themselves, then the flow-on effect of that is tremendous. When you're achieving personal goals with a positive mindset and are focusing on more than just your career, your friends and family are going to notice and some of that positivity will rub off on them.

My hope is that this book will spark that chain reaction and that you will be part of the ignition. I know it sounds a bit cheesy to say I want to make the world a better place. But over the years, I've worked with thousands of clients who have gone through their own Personal Revolutions and I've seen the positive impact on their lives, their friends and their families. So, I know that it's not just wishful thinking to say I want to make the world a better place. When people take control of their health and fitness, their lives and the people around them benefit.

So, who is this book for?

This book is for anyone who has been focusing on their career at the cost of their health and fitness. For anyone who has tried multiple times to get healthy, to feel good about themselves, to have the body and personal life they've always wanted, but who keeps failing. For anyone who looks in the mirror and hates what they see.

For anyone who's achieved a level of success and accomplishment at work, yet comes home and feels tired, unmotivated and unhealthy. For anyone who feels they aren't giving the best example to their children. For anyone who wants to lead the fit, healthy life they've always envisioned. For anyone who wants to learn how they can be the person they *want* to be, without sacrificing everything to get ahead in their career.

In this book, you'll discover a five-step process to help you achieve your own Personal Revolution. Here's a summary of the five steps:

- **Clarity:** Figure out your 'who', 'what', 'why' and 'how' to gain a deeper understanding of yourself and discover your short- and long-terms goals.
- **Measurement:** When you track it, you can improve it. Discover the metrics required to track and determine how you are improving and the results you are achieving.
- **Discipline:** Create positive habits and maintain them through strict yet achievable routines. These keep you accountable to yourself and the bigger picture, which is to live a balanced, high-performing life in all aspects.
- **Nutrition:** Eat healthy, live well, feel great. Only when you fill your body with the right ingredients, in the right amounts, can you achieve the physical and mental states you desire.
- **Exercise:** Movement is the foundation of life. To run on all cylinders and remain injury free, you need to be exerting yourself physically by working out and using different movement patterns.

As you read this book and uncover the five-step process to achieving your Personal Revolution, you will be taken on quite the personal journey. Some of the steps require you to dedicate time to sit and work through some exercises. These need to be taken seriously and given priority if you are to truly succeed at taking back your health and fitness.

Although it may only take you a few days to read through the book, I encourage you to take your time and implement the steps slowly over a six-week period. If you signed up for my one-on-one coaching programs or small group workshops, we would take six weeks or longer to go through the steps. So trust me, I'm saying this because I know it takes that long. One of the biggest mistakes you could make is thinking that you could change your life and take control of your routine, diet, workouts and goals within a week or two.

I'm not saying this to discourage you. But from my fifteen years of experience, I can assure you that the reason so many people attempt to change their life but give up after a few weeks is because they try to change everything at once. My suggestion to you is to read right through the book first, so that you understand all the concepts, and get a feel for the journey you are about to take. Then, using the resources I'll share with you, you can set up your own Personal Revolution and finally take control of your fitness and health.

Sound good? Great – let's get started!

FIVE RULES TO WIN YOUR PERSONAL REVOLUTION

I'm excited to share my five-step process for your Personal Revolution. But before I do, there are five key rules you need to apply before you start your journey to take back your health and fitness.

As you may have discovered, this journey is a lot more complicated than simply hiring a trainer and going on a diet. It requires a strategic battle plan, shaped by a series of rules designed to keep you on track and help you achieve your goal. If you're determined to win your Personal Revolution, there are five rules you need to follow:

1. The 'take ownership of your life' rule
2. The '80%' rule
3. The 'no right way' rule
4. The 'I can actually do this' rule
5. The 'one night a week' rule

In this chapter, you'll discover what each rule entails, why it's important, and how best to follow it in order to maximize your chances of success.

THE 'TAKE OWNERSHIP OF YOUR LIFE' RULE

One of the biggest mistakes people make is not taking 100 per cent ownership of their life, particularly their wellbeing. I can't stress enough how important this rule is to achieve a Personal Revolution. If you don't follow this rule, I can guarantee that you won't permanently take control of your health and fitness, and that the stresses of work and life will consume you again after a while. You must take charge, you must want to change, and you must be willing to do the hard work.

I've lost count of the number of successful executives I've worked with over the years who've told me that they are too busy to work out, even though they really want to. Similarly, I've lost count of the number of times I've heard excuses like, 'I don't know how to cook, so I don't.' Or, 'I'm just not a disciplined person, so I can't get up early like you to work out.'

There is an old saying: 'You can lead a horse to water, but you can't make it drink.' I can give you all the tools, every diet, every workout, and more. You can even read right through this book and follow the five-step process exactly as it's laid out. But if you're doing it just because I tell you to do it, and you don't take ownership of each step along the way, eventually it will be too easy to just go back to the way things were. It's *your* life, after all. As much as I want you to be the best version of yourself – fit, healthy and happy – you have to want it more than me, and you've got to fight for it. Revolutions are hard to win. Those old bad habits aren't going to give up their seat on the throne easily.

PETER'S STORY

When one of my clients (let's call him Peter) started working with me, he was the vice president of a global advertising agency. He is in his fifties and has spent his entire life working hard, focusing on his career and moving his way up the corporate ladder. He has all the worldly 'success' markers one could want in life. The car, the house, the nice clothes, the six-figure pay cheque, and so on.

However, his personal life was in complete chaos. His workout schedule was completely unstructured, so he would miss more workouts than he would do, and he had a significant recreational drug problem. His mind was scattered from late-night pitches, twelve-hour days, and working to meet client deadlines. He was the poster child for the typical overworked, type A executives I see all the time. Pushing the limits of their career to get ahead, yet sacrificing their health and wellness to get there. Even though he had a trainer, and a chef delivering his meals, he had never really taken true ownership of his life and what was actually going on.

So when I started coaching him, it took me a while to get him to understand that just because he had hired me, I couldn't change his life for him. I could help him and show him the tools, but I couldn't actually do the personal work. Eventually, after a lot of resistance and pushback, I got him to a place where he was able to look in the mirror and take complete responsibility for his situation and ownership of his personal health.

He stopped his recreational drug habit, which meant he was able to sleep better, which meant he was able to commit to working out five days a week, which meant he was able to start seeing results, which meant he felt better about himself when he looked in the mirror, which gave him a sense of pride and achievement, which inspired him to start taking care of his neglected friendships, which made him happier, which made him evaluate his entire life, which prompted him to learn how to cook for himself, which gave him more ownership of his life, and so on and so on.

The point I'm trying to make is that without Peter taking complete ownership of his life, all the money thrown at his health and fitness would never have made the impact he wanted. In short, if he hadn't followed this crucial rule, he never would've won his Personal Revolution.

THE '80%' RULE

This rule is super important because, when it comes to attempting a Personal Revolution, most people don't abide by it. Yet without it, permanent change and success are almost impossible to achieve.

To explain this rule, I want you to think back to a time in your life when you or someone you know attempted to take control of their health and fitness. It's a new year, you're super motivated, and you're finally going to start working out properly and eating right. You're going to lose some weight, and at the same time start doing some yoga because your lower back hurts all the time. You're also going to start following that new diet, which requires you to throw all of your existing food out of the fridge, and at the same time start walking to work, which means you'll be getting up thirty minutes earlier every day.

You get the point.

Trying to do all of this at once is trying to do 100 per cent of everything all the time. How long do you think you can last at 100 per cent? From my experience, most people last six weeks – maybe eight if they have a trainer and have thrown a lot of money at them. After that, the motivation starts to drop off, something stressful happens at work, and you stop one of these new changes. Then it becomes like a house of cards, as everything else quickly falls away. Now you feel even worse about yourself. You feel like a failure – like you wasted your money and time trying to better yourself. 'Looking good' and 'feeling good' is just something you'll never get in life.

Then six or twelve months later – it may even be years later – you attempt the exact same process again, maybe this time at a different gym, on a different diet, because 'Last time I wasn't with a good trainer, and this new diet everyone is doing is way better.' And so, the cycle continues.

If you look at this graph of someone living optimally at 100 per cent for eight weeks, then back to zero per cent for six months and then back to 100 per cent for eight weeks, and so on, you get this wave effect over the course of five years of their life.

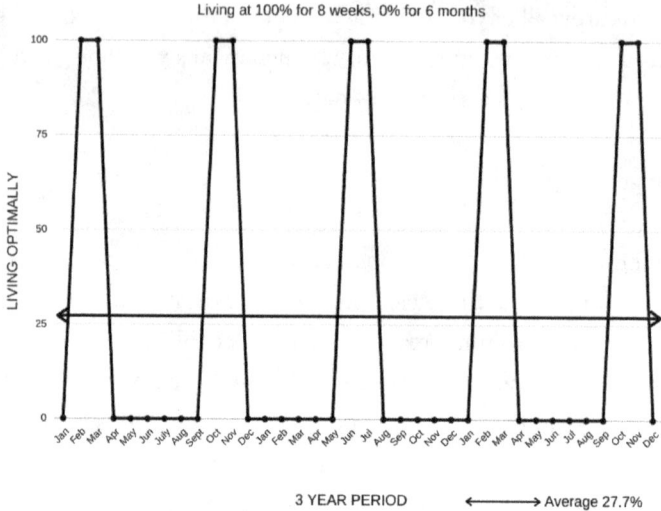

Let's just say, for argument's sake, that you were living at 100 per cent for eight weeks and then gave up and went back to your old ways for the next eight weeks, and then back to 100 per cent for eight weeks. You would be living your life at the best level you could for only fifty per cent of the time. Remember, I said most people go back to their old ways for months, if not years. So realistically, the average time spent doing everything right is probably only ten to twenty per cent.

This is where the eighty per cent rule comes into play. What if I told you that when it comes to everything I'm telling you to do in this book, you only need to do eighty per cent of it? So, when it comes to incorporating a morning routine, just try and do it Monday to Friday, and enjoy a sleep-in on the weekend. Similarly, spend one day a week eating whatever you want.

Or let's say you try and work out five days a week, but some weeks you only manage to work out four times. In this instance, start to look at the big picture. For example, let's say you did really well for four weeks and then in the fifth week things at work get really insane. You end up not working out at all, and you're eating junk food at the office to get through the week. Knowing that you're living your life with this eighty per cent rule in play means that, rather than feeling terrible and just giving up (like most people), you can say to yourself, 'You know what? Four out of five weeks isn't that bad. That's eighty per cent, so I'm good.' You feel in charge and still motivated because, unlike before, you're owning this situation and you know what to do.

You can see now that the person living by the eighty per cent rule will be ahead of the person living this wave of zero to 100 per cent, with an average of fifty per cent. (Remember, this number is so exaggerated, yet eighty per cent still beats it.)

Also, by keeping at eighty per cent over the long term, you get the benefit of compound interest, whereby your results just keep stacking up – pushing you even further ahead of the person living the wave effect. The longer you maintain this level of commitment, the easier and easier it becomes, and the more and more you solidify your results and progress as they keep building on top of each other. I've been doing this for so long now that even if I took two or three months off eating well and exercising, the moment I went back to it, I would bounce back to where I am now relatively quickly.

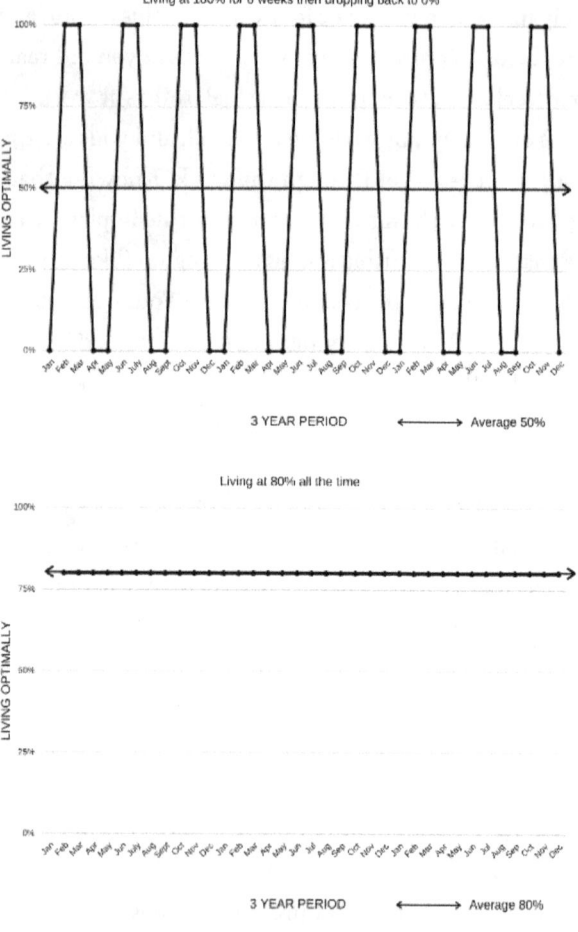

THE 'NO RIGHT WAY' RULE

This rule doesn't require a huge amount of explaining, but it's worth discussing because I see a lot of clients getting caught up on this. Instead of focusing on just embracing and implementing positive change, everyone is focused on figuring out the right way to do it first.

I've heard this plenty of times: 'I'm not going to start eating healthily because I don't know the right diet.' Or, 'I'll start working out when I find the best workout for me.' What I find is that the best diet or workout for me might not be the best diet for you, and that is okay. If you want to be a vegan and I want to be a carnivore, for example, then that's okay.

The key is to stick to the rules and principles laid out in this book. Whatever tools you end up using to help you win your Personal Revolution, be it intermittent fasting or extrinsic motivation systems (we will cover these later in the book), if they help you to get the results you want, and you can stick to this approach in the long term, then isn't that the right way?

Understanding and applying this rule also takes a lot of pressure off you, because life changes and you need to be adaptable. If you're rigid and stuck on a certain routine, then when you get thrown off it, you don't know what to do, and you end up going back to doing nothing.

While I was working for a gym as the head trainer and group fitness manager, it came under financial stress and closed overnight, leaving hundreds of members without a gym. Because I had been there for a number of years and I lived in the area, I would bump into these members all the time on the streets and I would ask them, 'Where are you working out now?' You wouldn't believe the number of them who simply stopped working out. In their minds, they had created this routine and system around going to that particular gym, doing particular classes, and seeing particular people while they worked out. Now that the 'right way' of looking after themselves was gone, they just did nothing.

Maybe that's happened to you before – you moved to a new house, or your work schedule changed, and all of a sudden your routine changed, too. As a result, you end up not doing anything because you're stuck in your old ways. If you're serious about winning your Personal Revolution, you must understand that there's no 'right way' to live a happy and healthy lifestyle.

THE 'I CAN ACTUALLY DO THIS' RULE

You want a Personal Revolution? You want to finally feel good, look good, and like what you see? Then say it: 'I can actually do this!' I don't care if you've tried to change your life a hundred times before reading this book. Or maybe you've *never* tried because you think you can't.

If you're a human being, you have the capacity to not only be successful at work, but also have the body you want, live pain free and not feel your age. But you have to back yourself. If you're going to join a fitness class, don't go there saying, 'I don't think I can do this class – it's too hard.' Do you think you'll struggle in that class? One hundred per cent. If you go in saying, 'I can actually do this – I'll go at my own pace, but I've got this', chances are you will get through that class and think, 'Actually, that wasn't too bad at all.'

I can tell you, from my experience of instructing over 1,000 fitness classes, that the people who come in with the right mindset and attitude are the ones who stay around long term. Like most things in life, going into any new situation with a positive mindset is going to make the situation a lot better for you, and everyone around you.

When you go into a fitness class thinking, 'I can actually do this', the other people in the class can feel your energy, they can tell that you are there with a positive attitude, and they are more likely to talk to you and connect with you. I think we all would rather be around someone who is positive and determined than someone who's negative and defeatist.

The flow-on effect of this small change in mindset is profound. Imagine you're trying to embark on a Personal Revolution, and you've been trying to add exercise to your weekly routine for years. You eventually try a fitness class for the first time. You go with a positive mindset, and some cool people welcome you in the class. You feel accepted and comfortable, which makes you want to go again and again (which you do). Each time, you talk to more people, feel a little bit more comfortable, and ultimately become hooked.

Now you go all the time. You've made friends, and those friends encourage you to join their lunch club. You don't really know how to cook, but you think 'I can actually do this', so you join. Now you're learning to cook, eating healthily, feeling great. The point I'm trying to make is that by having a positive mindset, people will be more likely to accept you and help you, which means you're more likely to stick to the new habits you're trying to create, which means you're more likely to achieve life-changing results, becoming that better version of yourself you've been seeking for so long.

THE 'ONE NIGHT A WEEK' RULE

This is more of a literal rule than some of the others, which are more guidelines or principles to follow. It almost falls under the eighty per cent rule because it's the same principle, but it's more specific.

The 'one night a week' rule means doing or eating something you want one night a week. I've religiously followed this rule for over ten years by eating pizza every Friday night. I don't think any of us should deprive ourselves of things that we like. Life is too short, and I believe you should enjoy everything in moderation. So, I never tell any of my clients to not eat pizza, ice cream, burgers, or whatever their vices are.

Remember, you are in this for the long game; the changes you are making are meant to be permanent. If I told you that for the next eight weeks I want you to consume no sugar, no junk food and no alcohol, I know you have enough willpower to make it through those eight weeks. You're probably going to lose a lot of fat, too, and see some big improvements in your body. But how miserable are you going to be? I've done it before and, even for me, it was really tough, and I didn't enjoy life while I was doing it.

Also, what do you think happens when the eight weeks are up? You're going to binge on all those things for the next few weeks, since you've been depriving yourself of them entirely. Now guess what happens to the results you've just achieved? You guessed it. They are gone, and you've even added more fat than you lost in the first place. Now you feel ten times worse about yourself than you did eight weeks ago, and now you're *never* going to try to get in shape again.

So back to me and my pizza night. I absolutely love pizza – I could eat it all the time. But let's face it. You and I both know that pizza isn't the best thing for you. It's also one of the most convenient foods to order when you're too tired to cook or you forget to buy groceries. So, I know myself well enough that I don't want the temptation of ordering a pizza whenever the thought crosses my mind, so I set the rule that I eat pizza every Friday night. Here is what happens when I put this rule in place:

- I have something to look forward to every week.
- Any time I think about ordering a pizza any other night, I remember I'm having pizza on Friday and there is no way I want to eat pizza twice a week.
- I've added a small layer of structure to my weekly routine.
- I never feel guilty for sitting down and eating pizza.
- I'm in charge of my eating habits, as I'm thinking about the big picture rather than just getting through each day.
- I'm less likely to eat other forms of junk food during the week.

In recent years, I've also applied this rule by drinking some alcohol every Wednesday night. I call it Whisky Wednesday, whereby I have a small pour of bourbon or some other spirit after dinner. I do it for the exact same reasons mentioned earlier. It gives me something to look forward to, means I'm less likely to drink any other night of the week, and so on.

Before I put this rule in place, there were times in my life, particularly when I was tired or feeling burnt out, when I would come home and have one beer. Then it becomes the following night as well, then it becomes two beers a night and then, before I know it, I'm drinking a couple of beers on Wednesday, Thursday, Friday and Saturday night. It's too easy to slide into a habit like that, so, by enjoying a small pour once a week, I never go down that path of drinking night after night.

Obviously, these examples are very specific to me and my 'vices'. I'm not saying that you have to implement them for yourself, but if they resonate with you then by all means go for it. Spend some time thinking about what habits or things in your life you're struggling to keep under control and apply this rule. It could even be applied to something like only working late at the office once a week. If you have a problem with staying back in the office all the time, and you never have time to work out, then allocate one workday when you stay back to work. Then give yourself time on other nights to go to the gym. You will be surprised how effective this rule is.

CHAPTER SUMMARY

Deep down, there is a little anarchist running around inside of your mind, thinking they can just do and eat whatever they want. Try and control that little terror without any rules and see how you go. Chances are, he or she has been running free and easy, and you've bounced from week to week, trying (unsuccessfully) to stay on some sort of track.

In order to put a stop to this and set you on course to win your Personal Revolution, you need some simple guidelines. With that in mind, here's a quick recap of the five rules outlined in this chapter. As you move through the various steps of the Personal Revolution process, you can refer back to these rules as and when necessary.

Rule number one: Take ownership of your life

It's your life, not mine. I've turned plenty of clients away in the past because I just know they aren't truly taking ownership of their life yet. Don't throw money at me, thinking that's it's 'problem solved'. You still have to do the work.

Rule number two: Eighty per cent is good enough

I know you like to ace tests and come first in your class, but, unless you plan on becoming a fitness model, you aren't going to last long trying to operate at 100 per cent with regard to health and fitness. Lower the bar, feel good if you're nailing eighty per cent of what you want, and remember you are playing the long game now. I want you to be fit for life, not just two months each year before summer so you can fit into your bathing suit.

Rule number three: There's no right way – what works for me might not work for you!

There is no right way. It's about the effort and the act of trying to live a better and healthier life. I might love fasting; you might hate it. You might love running; I might hate it. I don't have to run and you don't have to fast to achieve the results we want. The worst mistake you could make is thinking that it's 'my way or the highway'. Figure out what works best for you.

Rule number four: You can *actually* do this!

Stop believing this idea that you can't be fit, you can't lose weight, and you can't be happy with yourself. I can almost guarantee I've had clients in worse shape than you, who doubted themselves more than you might be doubting yourself right now. So if you have that little voice in the back of your head telling you that you can't do this, and you can't last more than a month living healthy, it's time to block that voice out. If you're truly ready for a Personal Revolution, now is the time to have one.

Rule number five: Identify your 'one night a week' treat and enjoy it

Sometimes the best way to solve a 'problem' is to own it, face it, accept it, reframe it, and turn it into something you have control over. If eating sugar is a problem for you, then instead of just depriving yourself of it for as long as you can until you finally break, dedicate one night a week to eating as much of it as you like. Just like my Friday pizza night, figure out what your 'one night a week' treat is and enjoy it. I can tell you that after ten years of doing this, I still love waking up every Friday morning, knowing what I get to eat for dinner that night.

> Now that you understand the rules of engagement and how they can help you win your Personal Revolution, it's time to consider the preparation required before you rise up and take back your life. That's the focus of chapters two, three and four.

2

CLARITY, PART 1

It's now time to start examining the five-step process to achieve your Personal Revolution. As you know, the first two steps are Clarity and Measure. These two steps are absolutely essential to successfully win this fight. However, they're often the two steps that most people never think about, and definitely don't take seriously.

I would argue that step one, Clarity, is the most important step, so please read through it slowly and carefully. It's important to really absorb what I am about to share with you, because this is where your Personal Revolution starts to take shape. We are going to create that spark; that 'aha!' moment that changes everything for you. It's going to be a game-changer as you progress further along your journey. There's a lot to cover, so step one is spread across two chapters (this one and the next). In this chapter, we'll focus on you as a person, looking specifically at your 'who', 'what', 'why' and 'how'.

IDENTIFYING WHO YOU ARE

Think back throughout history to some of the most well-known revolutionaries. Names like Che Guevara and Mahatma Gandhi are among the first names that come to mind. Do you think they had a clear sense of their identity and what they were fighting for? They couldn't have been clearer.

They could clearly define what their views and beliefs were, they could tell you exactly what their vision for the future was, they could tell you the purpose of their vision, and they had a clear strategy of how they were going to achieve their revolution. They were driven by long-term goals and a higher purpose, regardless of the consequences. Gandhi spent five years in jail for his revolution. However, his clarity on who he was and what he believed in was clear and strong – so much so that he was able to change history.

So, who are you? What do you want from your personal life? Are you crystal clear on your vision of your physical health and lifestyle outside of your career? Have you ever stopped for a moment to really think about it? I'm asking these deeper questions so that when things get chaotic in your life, and you start to feel yourself falling off the health and fitness wagon again, you can remind yourself of the bigger picture and why you're even doing all this in the first place. If Gandhi hadn't been deeply focused on – and committed to – his bigger picture, after a few cold, sleepless nights in jail he may have simply given up.

Time and time again, I'll sit down to a consultation with a client and I will ask them to explain what company they work for, what they do there – basically a 'who, what, why, how' of their career. Every person goes straight into this exciting, well-thought-out pitch about what their company does, what their role is, why they do what they do, what their goals are, and so on. It's actually surprising sometimes how much clarity they have around their career.

Then I will ask, 'Okay, forget about your career for a moment. Who are you as a person? What are your goals? How do you envision yourself?' Instantly you can feel the change in emotion. The client will shift in the chair, and their shoulders slump just slightly. They don't really know what to say. Most people say something along the lines of wanting to be healthy or wanting to lose weight or gain muscle. Other times, it's about not wanting to feel their age anymore or fix some sort of injury. These are all very short-term answers – 'I have a problem and I need to fix it.' If I pull the layers back a bit more, most people have no game plan or vision for themselves, other than being successful at work.

I'm now going to share with you a simple but highly effective exercise. You'll need to give yourself some time to sit down and take it seriously. If you answer these next four questions, you will gain the clarity you need to win your Personal Revolution, and live a healthy, active life.

WHAT ARE YOUR VIEWS AND BELIEFS?

Most people have never stopped and truly examined their beliefs. They've just accepted whatever beliefs were imprinted on them, either through their own mind or passed on by others. The important thing to understand is that some of these beliefs may be good and serving you well, while others may, in fact, be sabotaging your health.

Before we go any further, what is a belief? What does a view – particularly a view about yourself – even mean? A belief is defined as 'an acceptance that a statement is true or that something exists.' Notice the use of the word 'acceptance'? Beliefs are not facts. Beliefs or views are the assumptions you believe are true. They come from real life experience – because what you believe, you experience. You may think that your experiences are the reality of your life, when in fact it's your beliefs that govern your experiences.

This is so important to understand because your beliefs act as a filter to the outside world. You don't collect information that makes you form new beliefs; you collect information that supports the beliefs you already have. This means that if you believe that working out is too hard for you, then every time you attempt to work out – be it jogging, fitness classes, weight lifting or even yoga – you will find reasons to believe that these activities are too hard for you to do.

For you to understand who you are, you need to understand what your beliefs are. Your beliefs control your behaviours, so you need to make sure that what you truly believe is powerful enough to impact your daily choices. Likewise, if you have any negative beliefs about yourself, it's time to dump those in the garbage and realign yourself with beliefs that move you. Some common negative beliefs are statements like:

- 'I can never look good; I've always been overweight.'
- 'I'm just not the physical type.'
- 'I don't deserve to be in amazing shape.'
- 'No one will ever like me for my body.'

Can you see how any negative beliefs you may have are controlling your behaviour? A simple statement like 'I'm not the physical type' would be enough to keep most people out of the gym. Or a statement like 'I've always been overweight; it's just who I am' would be enough to stop someone from taking care of their diet. Spend some time thinking about what views and beliefs you're holding on to. If they are negative, scrap them, and remind yourself of some positive beliefs you do have. Chances are you've just forgotten, or never stopped to realize, that you do actually believe statements like these:

- 'Nothing in my life is more important than my health and fitness.'
- 'I believe I'm in control of my physical health and wellbeing.'
- 'I can choose to slow down my body's aging process.'
- 'I can look and feel however I want.'

Read over those statements three times and think about how you're feeling. Do you feel even slightly inspired? If you don't believe them at all, then read over them ten times more until you do. Even better, take some time to write down some personalized statements you can get behind. What are your positive views and belief statements around your health and fitness? To help spark some ideas, here is my belief statement.

JAY'S BELIEF STATEMENT

'I believe that I have always been in control of my body and how I look and feel. My health and fitness is the most important aspect of my life, as it is the fundamental basis for everything else in it. I believe that I am capable of unlocking its full potential. My health and fitness is one of the biggest strengths and assets I own. I can look and feel however I want. I can move and function however I want. I can live a longer and more fulfilling life when I focus on my health and fitness!

Make sure you pick beliefs that will move you at a deeper level. The next part of this exercise is to figure out exactly how you envision yourself to be if you were the best version of yourself, physically and mentally. Your vision for yourself will come to fruition based on your beliefs, so pick wisely.

There isn't a single aspect of your life that your physical health does not affect. It's connected to how you feel emotionally, the way you think, the way you view yourself, the way others view you, and more. Everything in your life is affected by your health and fitness.

You can change your life right now, so take it seriously. When you start believing right now that nothing is more important than your health and fitness, things will change. And if you believe you're in control and you have the ability to look after yourself, those beliefs will transform the way you think about your health and fitness from now on.

And don't just say it. You need to truly believe it!

WHAT IS YOUR VISION FOR YOURSELF?

This part of the book is, in my opinion, the most exciting and fun to read, as you get to use your imagination and dream up a version of yourself that you may have never thought about before. You've spent some time thinking about your beliefs and hopefully you're in the process of removing any negative ones. Now is the time to get creative. It's time to think about exactly the kind of person you want to be in relation to your health and fitness. This is a Personal Revolution, after all. No one fought a revolution to simply change a couple of minor things. We are overthrowing it all here for a better version of you and a completely different way of doing things.

A clear understanding or vision of yourself helps you to become who you want to be and to achieve your personal goals. A vision that is clear will open your mind to the endless possibilities of the future. A vision for yourself is simply a target. Think of it like a business target. Every company has a vision it is working toward – a future version of the company it is trying to achieve. Why shouldn't the same apply to you? If you do not have a vision of who you want to be, how you want to succeed or what you want out of life, you begin to lack drive and your life becomes just a series of events. Why go to the gym or eat well if you have no real reason to improve yourself?

Regardless of what is going on at work or what challenges are presenting themselves, a strong vision helps you know what you're doing and why you are doing it. Getting up at 6:00 a.m. to go to the gym becomes that little bit easier if you're focusing on a bigger picture, rather than just going to the gym because you think you have to.

It's important to have a vision in every aspect of your life, but particularly in your personal health and fitness. This is for life. Having optimal health needs to span a lifetime, not just three months, so you better create a powerful vision for yourself that will transcend not months, not years, but decades.

Writing down a version of yourself that you want to become is not only foretelling but also inspirational. Imagine having a clear and perfect understanding of who and what you want to become. The steps to becoming that will become clearer, as there is a path now laid out in front of you to follow. It's like a fortune teller just whispered your future in your ear and all you need to do is follow the signs.

There is something magical about seeing words on a piece of paper that describe this upgraded version of yourself – a version you can only imagine right now. So, what do you want for yourself? Close your eyes and imagine the person you see before you. If you could have or be anything you wanted in this part of your life, what would it be?

Can you imagine yourself lean and fit?

What about big and muscular?

Do you want to live for a long time with perfect health?

Do you want the same sense of pride in your personal life as you have in your professional life?

Whatever it is, write it down.

To give you an idea, I'll share with you what's written on my vision statement. My vision will be different from yours, of course. Remember, we are all on a different journey and path. However, I'm happy to share mine so you can see what I mean by an actual statement of who and what you want to become.

JAY'S VISION STATEMENT

'My vision of myself is to be in fitness-model shape for the rest of my life. I want to be a billboard for fitness wherever I go. I want to have ripped abs, a tapered back and a small waist all the time. I see myself as someone who can run fast and run long distances. I can do yoga, fight, crawl, swim, and move in any direction.

'I live with no pain, or self-doubt in my abilities to participate in any physical activity. I see my wife being physically attracted to me for the rest of my life. My health and fitness are part of my identity, and I want people to be inspired by that. I am going to live for as long as I can, and be injury and sickness free.'

When I read that, I see all these little markers in there that give me inspiration for what I need to be doing in my life. For example, if I want to have 'ripped abs, a tapered back and a small waist', that means I need to be paying close attention to my diet, because to have those three things I need to be very lean. If I want to 'run fast and long distances', that means I better be including running in my life. If I can 'do yoga, fight, crawl, swim, and move in any direction', then guess what? I better be doing yoga, boxing, swimming and movement training as part of my workout routines, or I'm not going to be the person I envision myself to be.

Can you see how, by spending some time writing down a few paragraphs detailing who I want to be, I can use it to reverse engineer what I should be doing? And if I start doing those things, I can actually be the person I want to be.

It's funny how, sometimes, the simplest things can end up being the most powerful sparks that can change your whole direction in life. Maybe you envision yourself being able to keep up with your kids playing sports. By writing that down, a light bulb has just turned on. You aren't even spending time *now* playing sports with your kids, so you're going to start doing that. The better version of you can start as soon as you put this book down.

Now that we've covered the 'who' and the 'what', it's time to move into the 'why'.

WHY DO YOU WANT TO CHANGE?

The truth of the matter is that most people know how to work out and how to look after themselves. Deep down you know, 'If I work out and eat better, I'm going to look and feel better.' We all know these fundamental truths. But if you're not sure *why* you want to make these changes, you won't get very far. If your 'why' is weak, that's why you aren't living the fit and healthy life you want – or why you're not able to stick to it.

If I asked you, 'Why do you want to make more money?', or,

'Why do you work so much?', you could give me a dozen reasons straightaway as to why your career and making money are important to you. In other words, you most likely have some pretty strong clarity around why you do what you do in the financial and career aspects of your life.

So, why do you want to be fit and healthy? If you cared as much about it as you do about making money, do you think you would struggle to be fit and healthy? There are some people out there who legitimately don't care about their body or their health. They are happy to eat junk food, never work out, and don't look after themselves. It's sad, but it's their life and their body. I have people like that in my own life and I really worry about them as they get older, as it's going to get tougher for them.

Maybe there's a little part of you, or a big part, that, up until this point, hasn't really cared about your health and wellbeing. That's a reality you're here to break. Well, good for you. It's not easy and, unfortunately, you're going to have to go a little bit deeper into the pain of that reality to come out the other side with a purpose and a 'why' that will be unbreakable as you move forward from this point. A strong enough purpose will wipe out all excuses.

Firstly, you need to acknowledge the pain that not looking after yourself is causing you. You've got to go deep; this is between you and yourself. I can't help you with this part. However, here are some questions to help you acknowledge any pain or discomfort you may be feeling:

- How do you feel when you look in the mirror?
- What's the cost of not looking after yourself?

- What does your future look like?
- If you keep doing what you're doing, what's your quality of life going to be? Is your body going to start falling apart? Are you more likely to get sick and/or injured?
- Think about your particular situation. For example: If I keep working fourteen-hour days with only five hours' sleep each night, what will happen to me? What is happening to me now?
- Are you setting a good example for your kids?
- How do you feel knowing that as successful as you are in other areas of your life, this part is a failure?
- Why aren't you committed to being the best version of yourself?

These are tough questions, I know, and it's really hard to admit to yourself if any of these are true. However, the only way you are going to make permanent changes in your life is to face all these hard questions head on and deal with the reality of your current situation.

To help you do this, write down all the negative things that will happen or continue to happen if you *don't* change your behaviour. What does your life look like? I'm guessing it's not a nice list of emotions, feelings and outcomes. But this is your truth. Sorry, I can't sugar-coat it in any way or spin it to make it look good.

Don't worry. It gets better, I promise. Take that horrible list of negative things and reverse them all to be positive if you *do* change your behaviour. What will you gain if you take control of your health and fitness and become the person you want to become? Here are some questions to help get you started:

- How will you feel when you look in the mirror?
- What do you gain from looking after yourself?
- What does your future look like now?
- What does your quality of life look like?
- Will you be more likely to find a partner?
- Will you live longer for your children?
- Would you be even more successful at work, now that you're healthy, fit and optimized?

I'm guessing this list is now looking pretty awesome. I'm guessing this list of things you will gain is pretty exciting. I'm guessing you've got enough reasons now to create a strong enough 'why' for yourself. Imagine if you have all those new feelings, emotions and outcomes in your life just by dedicating the time to looking after yourself. Is it worth having all that negativity in your life simply by not looking after yourself, when you could have immense positivity in your life instead? It's hard to turn your back on that once you see it.

You need to dig deep into the pain you're suffering, and the price you're paying, by not looking after yourself. Then think about the new you that's on the other side of a change in your behaviour. Once you do this, you will be able to break any unhealthy habit and live the life you want to.

I'll share with you my 'why' statement, although it's specific to me. Remember, you have to go through this process on your own. However, I want to show you what keeps me motivated and driven even when I don't want to go to the gym, or eat in a way that keeps me looking and feeling my best.

JAY'S 'WHY' STATEMENT

'My "why" is to be a shining example of all the benefits a healthy and super-fit lifestyle can bring to someone's life. I want to be in incredible shape for my wife so that we will be attracted to each other for the rest of our lives. I can explore new and interesting techniques for being healthy and fit, and share that information with my friends and family. I can extend my life by many years by staying in the best shape, physically and mentally, possible.

'I want to be able to keep up with all the children in my life as they grow older, and as I do. I want to be known as the uncle who cannot be beaten, who can keep up with anything they do, so I can show them a good example of how to live their own lives. This is why I prioritize my health and fitness over anything else in my life. Because I know if I do, I will be more successful, I'll feel better, I'll have more opportunities, and I will have a better quality of life for as long as I live.'

HOW ARE YOU GOING TO ACHIEVE YOUR VISION?

There are two universal things that are fundamental to looking after your body and your health. Those two things are some sort of nutritional plan and some sort of exercise plan. All of us need to have at least these two things in place. I'll be going into detail about these two plans later, in chapters six and seven, as they are both part of the five-step Personal Revolution process.

So, without going into great detail on either topic (in an effort to avoid repeating myself later), this exercise is designed to help you create an outlining strategy that you can start to put into place. Now that you've spent some time getting crystal clear on why you need to look after yourself, you need a strategy or battle plan to achieve that.

We've talked about creating a battle plan for winning your Personal Revolution. Well, the time for that is now. *How* are you going to be in the best shape possible? *How* are you going to get the right kind of food into you? *How* are you going to find time to get more sleep, or time to work out?

You need to physically write out a strategy plan, so that you see it in front of you. This strategy plan needs to cover everything you can think of that will help you achieve your vision of yourself. It needs to scope out beyond just working out and eating well. You're aiming now for the best possible version of you: healthy, fit and in shape. What is it going to take to get that?

You may not have all the answers on how to do that just yet, so perhaps the first thing on your list is to implement everything I'm teaching you in this book. Then the next thing is to take some cooking lessons because you don't know how to cook. Let me give you my 'how' plan as an example, as I think reading one will give you some clarity on what you need to do. Again, remember this 'how' is specific to what I want in *my* life, so don't just copy it, but feel free to use some of it if you like it and it resonates with you.

JAY'S STRATEGY PLAN

'To live as a highly physical and optimal person, I need to have a morning, evening and daily ritual that becomes part of my everyday routine. I need to eat well, sleep well, train hard and ensure that my mind is always taken care of.

'I need to pencil time in my calendar for other physical activities, such as movement, yoga, swimming and running, for example, as these will help me to build the functional and rounded physical abilities I need to live the life I want.

'My physical and healthy lifestyle needs to include body work on a regular basis, such as massage, chiro, acupuncture and stretching. I will pencil these into my schedule to ensure I never miss an appointment. I will fast several times a year to allow my body and organs to rest and regenerate. I will always be up to date with the latest breakthroughs within this part of my life to make sure I am optimizing myself with the best techniques and routines.'

Can you see how I've created a plan to include all the things I want to be in my vision statement? All I need to do now is follow this plan to the best of my abilities and, over time, I will become the person I want to be.

Some of those strategies are quite simple, yet they changed my life after I implemented them. For example, for many years I was always getting massages at random times throughout the year. Yet often, when I would really need one, I couldn't get a booking.

I would spend weeks thinking that I needed to get a massage but wouldn't get around to booking one. One five-minute call with the massage studio and I was able to book in a massage every six weeks for an entire year. Done. Now I never have to worry about when I'm going to have a massage.

You would be surprised how easy it is to get some of your strategy in place, and how, after a few simple phone calls or emails, your whole life will completely change. How exciting is that?! Perhaps you're right at the very beginning of your journey and you've never worked out before, and you've never tried to follow a diet, or eat in a certain way. All of this sounds so daunting. Let me create a 'how' strategy plan for you to see how it might look.

YOUR HYPOTHETICAL STRATEGY PLAN

'In order for me to take control of my personal health and fitness, and to become the best version of myself, I am going to finish this book and attempt to implement the five-step Personal Revolution process outlined in it.

'Because I have never worked out before, I am going to ask some of my work colleagues if any of them work with a personal trainer near the office. If they do, and I am going to book in twelve sessions with them. I haven't looked after my body properly in years, so I am going to go to the doctor and get a physical check-up and make sure I don't have any preconditions or health issues I should be aware of.

'When I eat lunch at work, it is always unhealthy food, so I am going to start bringing my own lunch to work. I will buy five glass containers, do some research online to find some easy meal prep recipes I can follow, and make up some lunches for the week.'

A few simple paragraphs written out like this can instantly give you direction. Imagine taking that statement and following exactly what it said. Within a week, you could figure out where and how to work out. You would know what condition your body is in, and how to prepare healthy meals.

> **CHAPTER SUMMARY**
>
> This is powerful stuff – it really gets me going! The thought of you doing these exercises – and discovering your 'who', 'what', 'why' and 'how' – is so exciting.
>
> Please don't disregard this important work, as it really does shape the direction of your Personal Revolution. Time and time again, I've seen clients' lives change the moment they stop, sit down and get some clarity on their life. We've all got lost along the way at some point. It's time to get back to being the person you truly want to be.

3

CLARITY, PART 2

Now that you understand who you are, what your beliefs are, what you want, and how you're going to get it, let's take it one step further. In this chapter, which forms the second part of step one (Clarity), you'll figure out what kind of motivation works for you. You'll also discover the art of effective goal setting.

Both of these things are crucial components of your Personal Revolution, as they enable you to take full control of the journey – and give you the best chance of success. Without them, you risk losing motivation and focus, which may lead you to give up altogether. So, to ensure that doesn't happen, please make sure you read this chapter carefully.

UNDERSTANDING WHAT MOTIVATES YOU

There are two types of motivation: intrinsic and extrinsic. Intrinsic motivation occurs when people are motivated by internal rewards. For example, 'I always work out because I love the feeling of self-improvement.' Extrinsic motivation occurs in people who are driven by the thought of external rewards, such as money or objects. For example, 'I always work out because I love the looks people give me when they see I'm in shape.'

There are different types of motivation that sit under each of these two broader categories, and we will go through a couple of examples that are most common when it comes to sticking to a fitness or self-improvement program. Understanding what kind of motivation works for you is really important because then you can figure out what motivational triggers work for you.

Are You Financially Motivated?

If you spend money on something, are you guaranteed to fulfill that commitment because it costs you something? In other words, the thought of wasting that money overrides the desire to not do it. Personally, I know I am highly motivated by that, which means if I want to achieve something, or do something, I need to pay for it in advance so that I'm 100 per cent committed to it.

For example, I paid upfront for a fitness show the moment I decided I wanted to participate so that I was forced train and diet for it. There was no way I was going to throw away that entry fee.

Are You Completion and Process Motivated?

Does completing a to-do list motivate you? Is the journey itself often the reward, not just the desired outcome?

If that's the case, then create a health and wellness checklist, or create a daily calendar, which includes hitting your calories, doing your workout, doing your morning routine, and so on. Give yourself a gold star each day you cross off that checklist. This is such a simple solution to keep you motivated, if you're the kind of person this will work for.

Are You Motivated by Gifts and Rewards?

If your biggest source of motivation is the prospect of gifts and rewards, create a reward system for yourself. Here are some great examples that either my clients or I have used to stay motivated and on track:

- If I don't eat takeaway food all week, I get to eat pizza on Friday night.
- If I work out four days a week for a whole month, I will buy myself a new workout outfit.
- If I lose fifteen pounds in six weeks, I will book myself a day at the spa or a weekend away.
- If I don't drink alcohol for a whole month, I will buy myself a bottle of expensive champagne and enjoy it as a reward.
- If I meal prep my lunches for four days, on Friday I get to order lunch from my favourite place.

If this is you, then look at your goals and vision for yourself, and set up a whole reward system around them to help you stay on track. We don't need to pretend that most of us aren't motivated in this way. At the end of the day, we're just big kids who still need to be bribed with candy to do our homework.

Are You Socially Motivated?

If you make commitments or plans with friends and family, are you more likely to stick to those plans for fear of letting people down? If someone asks you how certain things are going, do you feel bad if you haven't been doing those things?

On the flip side, do you feel motivated when people ask how you're doing and you can share with them your progress? If that is the case, then hiring a trainer and making yourself accountable to them might be a good idea. Another idea is to involve some of your friends or family in your journey – again, to keep you accountable.

Be Honest With Yourself

Each person is unique. What works for some people doesn't work for others, so you have to be truly honest with yourself and spend some time considering what will actually motivate you. There is nothing wrong with being honest with yourself and saying, 'If I can achieve the goals I have set out for myself for the next three months, I'm going to go buy myself a new outfit and I'm going to love it!' If that is the only thing that will motivate you, then do it.

FRIENDS AND FAMILY: HELPING OR HINDERING?

This is a tough subject to talk about, but I think it is important to address because the people in your life could be holding you back from living the life that you want. If your colleagues around you at work are unhealthy and are making poor health choices, then it's going to be hard to maintain the discipline required to look after yourself. It's even harder if your friends and family are the same. What's worse is that they could even be subconsciously trying to sabotage your efforts.

Have you noticed how, whenever you say you're trying to eat better, all of a sudden everyone around you is offering you some sort of sugary treat? In order to stay motivated and win your Personal Revolution, you need to take a close look at your network of friends and family. How much are they helping or hindering you?

If none of your friends are working out, eating healthily, or looking after themselves, then I know you're fighting an uphill battle trying to stay on track. If you have people in your life that you know are pulling you backwards, then you need to really spend some time thinking about how you can manage them and their effect on your life.

It's a lot easier to go out with a friend who is also trying to eat healthily, as opposed to someone who doesn't care and always suggests eating a burger. If achieving this life vision you have for yourself is really a priority for you, then you need to have a conversation with these people and explain how important it is to you. If they aren't interested or fail to show any support, then you need to modify how they fit into your life.

I've been through this and it's tough. I've got friends who love to drink all the time, for example. I used to enjoy drinking a lot in my twenties, but now I don't want to. These friends always want to drink, so now I make sure that I really only see them for lunch or for organized events. I don't hang out with them as regularly anymore, because I don't want to be drinking with them all the time. It can be hard changing some of your relationships. I've even had to remove myself from friendships because they were too much of a negative influence on me and my life goals.

ALISON'S STORY

I worked with a lady called Alison, who worked as a mortgage director in a major bank here in Toronto. She had some serious goals to change her life by losing some weight and living a much healthier life.

However, when she started bringing her own healthy lunches to work, instead of buying lunch every day, the other ladies she sat with would make subtle comments about her lunch being so healthy, and implying that she was better than they were. They would also constantly offer her a bite of their junk food or put sugary snacks down in front of her – another subtle suggestion to try and make her deviate from her goals.

She eventually had to stop eating lunch with them. She would go get coffee with them later in the day, or see them in other situations, but she removed herself from that negative situation in order to stay on track and ultimately win her Personal Revolution.

Of course, not everyone in your life will hinder your progress. On the contrary, many people may be cheering you on, so make sure that you are using the positive support group you have around you. Reach out to your friends and family, or close work colleagues, and tell them the journey you are on and the positive things you are trying to implement.

If you tell your friends that you've created a new morning routine and it is making a difference in your life and you're loving it, what are the chances that one of them will decide to try it too? Suddenly, you're now motivating each other. The flow-on effect of this is profound. For example, maybe now, instead of meeting up for drinks on the weekend, you are meeting up for a gym class. This is how it works. Positive actions create more positive actions.

THE ART OF EFFECTIVE GOAL SETTING

Goals and motivation are a bit like the chicken and the egg. I'm not really sure which one came first, but you need both in order to have one or the other. You can be highly motivated to change your life, but if you don't have a series of goals to work toward then that motivation isn't getting directed in the right places. Likewise, you could have all these goals, but if you aren't motivated then good luck achieving them. That is why goal setting is really important to keep you on track, and to keep you motivated in the short term and long term.

One very common mistake is to have either a short-term goal or a long-term goal and no roadmap in between. If your goal is very short term, then once you achieve it, what do you do next? It's easy to lose focus and fall back into old habits very quickly. Likewise, if your goal is very long term, then it will take a long time to feel like you are making any progress and, again, it's easy to lose focus. With the end result feeling so far away, you may decide it doesn't matter if you take some time off from working toward it.

Goal setting in your personal life has exactly the same structure as goal setting in business. Maybe if I switch the word 'goal' to 'target', that might resonate with you more. Chances are, whatever company you work for, you've got a series of targets broken up throughout the year, starting with an overall yearly target. Let's say it's five per cent profit growth. If this was the only target you had for an entire year, I'm guessing it would be pretty difficult to track the progress toward that goal.

Would anyone have a sense of urgency and push themselves all year to achieve that number? If you had a bad month, you wouldn't be too concerned because you have eleven months left to make things better. But before you know it, you've been under delivering for four or five months, and now it's impossible to make up the difference and achieve that target by the end of the year.

I know you're thinking, 'Yeah, Jay, I know how targets work and why we break them down into quarterly, monthly and fortnightly targets. It's what I do for a job, so get on with it.' Fair point – but I need to show you how this translates to your personal goal setting. Even the smartest CEOs I've worked with, ones in charge of companies pushing $100 million in yearly sales, with growth targets of ten per cent or more, come and tell me they've been trying to lose thirty pounds for the last couple of years and nothing has worked. I ask them what their game plan has been, and they say, 'Well, I've been working out and trying to eat better, and that's about it.'

Let's apply my example of having a yearly growth target with the goal to lose thirty pounds. Break up thirty pounds over a year, and that's two and a half pounds per month. If you haven't set your goal to lose two and a half pounds in the first month, and you don't lose the weight, you will think, 'It doesn't matter – it's just my first month. I'll do better next month.' The next month rolls on by, it's very busy and you miss a lot of your workouts, and you only lose one pound. Now you aren't feeling so great about yourself. In eight weeks, you've only lost one pound. How likely are you to give up now that you realize that losing thirty pounds – in this scenario – is pretty unlikely? You need to keep yourself accountable to your goals, just like in business.

Think of your life goals exactly as you would think of targets at work. If you want to win your Personal Revolution, you need your yearly goal, then you need your quarterly goals, and then you need your monthly goals. I even break it down to weekly goals and then right down to daily goals. It doesn't mean I have to live this militant life. It just means that I'm thinking about my personal goals, and being in control of my physical health and my wellbeing. This stops me getting caught between having a vague long-term goal and then trying to complete short-term goals which, once they end, take me back to square one.

AN EXAMPLE OF GOAL SETTING

Here is an example of how I would lay out my goals for the year:

Daily Goal: Do my morning routine and work out.

Weekly Goal: Work out a minimum of five times, and keep my weight between 168 and 173 pounds.

Monthly Goal: Reduce my body fat by one per cent.

Quarterly Goal: Compete in a fitness competition (book that now).

Half Yearly Goal: Run my first half marathon (commit to booking that now).

Yearly Goal: Be in better shape than I was last year.

Now, you can see I have a game plan that I'm thinking about all the time. It's specific and it requires me to commit to what I need to be doing. And as the year moves along, these goals will evolve. For example, once I've competed in my fitness competition, my quarterly goal would change to: 'Be able to run twenty kilometres', while my monthly goal would become: 'Complete a "learn how to run" program'. You get the idea.

KEEPING YOUR EYE ON YOUR NORTH STAR

This section might sound a little bit 'out there', but humour me and read it anyway. In chapter two, you completed a series of exercises to discover 'what' you truly want for yourself and 'why' you want it. I want you to bundle those two discoveries together and call them your North Star.

You're doing better than most people already by having thought through this stuff. But to win your Personal Revolution, you need to take it one step further. This vision and purpose have to be in the back of your mind at all times. You need to imagine it in front of you, like a North Star guiding your everyday choices. It's on your 'wall', like a company's core values.

Becoming the best version of yourself, physically and mentally, is a tough journey. You're going to get distracted and there will be times you fall off the wagon. Trust me! Over the twenty-plus years I've been working out, I can almost guarantee I've fallen off the wagon more times than you've got on it. So when you fall off and you aren't working out at all, and you aren't following any healthy eating habits, you need this clear objective, this

North Star, to remind you of why you're doing this in the first place. Say to yourself, 'I have the secret map that shows me the way. All I need to do is just follow that star and I'll get to where I want to be.'

It's time for you to start living your personal life with conviction and purpose. There is a better version of yourself waiting to be discovered, so focus on that vision and just start moving toward it. Remind yourself every day of that North Star, and think about how good you will feel when you look and feel like the person you imagine yourself to be.

JAY'S NORTH STAR

I still think about my North Star all the time. For me, being in shape is part of my career. If I wasn't in shape, my clients wouldn't take me seriously.

My North Star is envisioning myself much older, and still being able to run and jump around with my nieces and nephews. I'm able to pick any physical challenge and confidently attempt it. I have no aches and pains. I can move freely. I look twenty years younger than my age.

When I think about being that person, that motivates me to continually test myself with different workouts, it motivates me to take all my supplements and look after my diet, it motivates me to take care of my body and skin, and it motivates me to get enough sleep.

What is your North Star? Take some time to think about it and write it down somewhere. Live it, breathe it, become it.

CHAPTER SUMMARY

Imagine all this time you've been trying to motivate yourself with the wrong things. How great would it be to find motivation and have it actually stick this time?

Spend some time really thinking about what makes you tick. What kind of person are you? Does spending some money motivate you to go through with something? Does having a physical reward, like a new dress or workout shoes, motivate you to do something? There is nothing wrong with that – if that's what gets you going.

The worst thing you can do is try to motivate yourself with the wrong tools and then wonder why you still aren't staying committed to your goals. When those goals push you toward your North Star, everything is going to feel that much more dialled in. Write down your North Star and read it every day as part of your morning routine (more on this in chapter five). Read it until you know if off the top of your head. Get passionate about your life, your health and fitness, and your Personal Revolution.

4

MEASURE

Congratulations for completing parts one and two of Clarity – the first of the five steps in the Personal Revolution process. Now that you have some clarity around what it is you're working toward, it's time to move on to step two: 'Measure'.

When it comes to your Personal Revolution, you need to measure your success and track your progress. I'll use the revolution analogy to explain why this is important. At this stage, you know exactly what you're fighting for and why change must occur. You have an extremely specific battle plan, which you're going to use to win the fight. But how are you going to know if you truly succeed or not? How are you going to know if the battle plan you've created is working? That's the focus of this chapter.

IF YOU CAN'T MEASURE IT, YOU CAN'T IMPROVE IT

There is a great quote by Peter Drucker, who is regarded as the inventor of modern-day business management. He said, *'If you can't measure it, you can't improve it.'* Forget about business management – this couldn't apply more in your personal life, too. If you're trying to lose weight but you aren't regularly weighing yourself, then how are you going to know whether what you're doing is making you lose weight? In contrast, if you saw that your hard work was actually leading to results, how motivating is that going to be for you to keep doing what you're doing and lose more weight?

When I have a specific goal, be it fitness related, health related, or body related, I want to track the progress so I can make adjustments accordingly – before I waste time doing something that isn't working. There is nothing more satisfying for me than tracking my clients' results. Often, they come to me complaining that nothing happened over the last six weeks. They can't see or feel any changes, perhaps because they are always focusing on what still needs to change.

Once we redo their measurements, a specific set of markers that I will explain in the next section, they are always amazed at the results. Within seconds, they have gone from feeling completely negative to feeling extremely positive and pumped up for their next six-week program.

Tracking your progress also helps to break down your long-term goal into smaller chunks, so that the overall goal doesn't feel so daunting. I'll use the losing weight example again, since it will resonate with most people. If your long-term goal is to lose fifty pounds and you don't regularly track your progress, it's going to feel like an impossible task. Personally, I want to know each time I'm losing five pounds, so that I know I only have forty-five pounds left, or forty, or thirty-five, and so on. I'm also going to see that my goal is achievable. If every six weeks I track my results, and I'm losing five pounds over each six-week period, then I know that eventually I'm going to achieve my goal.

Also, by tracking my progress every six weeks and seeing that I'm losing five pounds over each six-week period, I can calculate how long it's going to take to achieve my goal of losing fifty pounds. Just do the math: fifty divided by five is ten. If I'm losing five pounds every six weeks, it will take sixty weeks to lose fifty pounds. That's over a year.

Tracking your progress will therefore set realistic expectations for you, as you can understand exactly how long it's going to take to achieve your goal, which makes it easier to stick to the plan. If you unrealistically think that losing fifty pounds is only going to take six months and you don't track your progress, and after six months you've only lost twenty-five pounds, you will think the whole thing has been a failure and you'll stop your program, even though you were actually on track. You just didn't realize it.

Another great reason to measure your success is to keep yourself accountable to your plan. There is something so simple about tracking your progress. Knowing that you have a measurement day coming up and you're going to be comparing your markers from before taps into your competitive side, because you want to beat your previous numbers and show yourself you did well.

Why do you think the sales department tracks its sales monthly, sometimes even weekly? It's always comparing the numbers to the previous month, and the previous year. It's motivated by the prospect of beating its previous best numbers. This drives the department to always strive to be better. Humans are competitive by nature. When we are given a metric that we can track, we naturally try to do better each time it's measured.

FOUR METRICS TO MEASURE YOUR SUCCESS

Now that you understand why it's so important to measure your success, I want to show you four different metrics you can use to do that. The first one I'm going to mention is obvious, and is what ninety-nine per cent of people use as a marker to measure themselves. It's your weight.

Weight

I would say one of the most common phrases I've heard, not just from my clients but even from friends and family, is, 'I'm trying to lose weight.' How many times has someone said that to you? How many times have you said that yourself? I've worked with dozens of people addicted to standing on their scale morning and night, every day of their lives. Join any diet challenge, or typical boot camp or fitness program, and the first thing they get you to do is stand on a scale so they can record your weight.

I'm not going to say that using weight as your metric to track your results is wrong. I'm just going to suggest that you shouldn't only be using weight as your marker. Imagine you went to the doctor for your yearly physical check-up, and all he did was put you on a scale and say, 'Well, you haven't gained any weight this year, so everything is fine.' Or 'You've lost quite a bit of weight this year, so it looks like you're doing great. Keep doing what you're doing.'

Wouldn't that be a bit troubling? What if you hadn't been doing anything different and you lost a bunch of weight? That could mean something was actually wrong with you. Wouldn't you want your blood work done, your eyesight checked, and so on? Just like the sales team at your company isn't just tracking sales (they're tracking returns, customer satisfaction, seasonal trends, and more), you need to be tracking multiple metrics to understand exactly how your progress is going.

Body Fat Percentage

One of my favourite markers to measure is body fat percentage, and I'll explain to you why. Firstly, let me explain what body fat percentage, or BFP, is. BFP is exactly what it sounds like – it is the percentage of your body that is made up of fat. Why BFP is so important is that no matter what you weigh, the higher percentage of body fat you have, the more likely you are to develop obesity-related diseases and suffer from other health issues, including heart disease, high blood pressure, stroke, and type 2 diabetes.

This means that two people who weigh exactly the same can have vastly different BFPs. One person can be healthy, fit and strong, while the other could be extremely unfit, unhealthy and at major risk of some serious diseases. It also means that by knowing someone's BFP and looking at their physical body, you can determine what kind of workout they should be doing.

For example, you could be quite small but have a very high BFP. In that case, I wouldn't be encouraging you to do a lot of cardio to try and burn off fat, as you would end up being just skin and bones. Instead, I would be telling you to gain some muscle. If you were large and overweight, and had a high BFP, then it would be the complete opposite – I would be encouraging you to try and lose some weight (aka fat).

It is often the case that I'll work with a client who isn't overweight – they might even be skinny and think that they are totally healthy – yet their BFP measurement is really high. It can be really eye-opening once you find out what that number is.

Body Circumference Measurements

The third metric I like to use to measure results is body circumference measurements, or BCM for short. This means taking measurements, with a tape measure, around different parts of your body, and then redoing those measurements at a later date. BCM is a tried and true way to measure results. It's particularly useful for someone who is trying to change their physical body, whether they're trying to lose extra fat or trying to gain muscle and overall size.

As I mentioned in the previous section, when someone is trying to change their body, they are looking at themselves every day in the mirror and focusing on all the negative parts. Based on this alone, it's extremely hard to tell if you have lost a couple of inches around your waist. By recording your BCM, you have proof in the numbers that explain exactly how and where your body has changed.

You can see now how frustrated you would be if you were only measuring your weight, and after six weeks it hadn't changed. However, if you had measured your BCM as well, and you had lost two inches around your waist and hips, then you wouldn't care about the scale at all.

Lifestyle

The last thing I like to measure is overall lifestyle improvement. I like to ask a series of questions that will get my clients to see some of the other positive improvements their Personal Revolution is giving them. It can be extremely frustrating for someone who is carrying a significant amount of extra weight to only lose a pound or two a week. However, the journey to losing that extra thirty pounds is going to take a while; it's a slow process.

It's easy to get disheartened and give up if you feel like nothing much is happening. You might think that only losing four pounds of fat in a six-week period is a failure. But if I asked you if you've been sleeping better and you have more energy, and you say yes, then to me that's a win.

There are so many other positive benefits of taking control of your health and fitness, but it's often hard to recognize them. We are all so focused on our appearance. Often, that's all we see. But if you want to win your Personal Revolution, you must take note of any positive improvements to your quality of life – not just the number on the scale, or how loose your jeans are.

> 'Measurement is the first step that leads to control and eventually to improvement.'
> – DOCTOR H. JAMES HARRINGTON

HOW TO TRACK YOUR PROGRESS

When it comes to tracking your progress, this is where the work you did in step one comes back into play. You need to be tracking in a way that is in alignment with your goals. So often I'm working with clients who are obsessed with weighing themselves two or three times a day, when their goals are actually to lose body fat and to maintain or even gain some muscle. If you aren't trying to lose weight, then why are you weighing yourself all the time? You're putting all this energy into tracking something that isn't even an indicator of the progress you should be making.

You may find it hard at first to figure out what you should be tracking, but the easiest thing to do is bring up your list of daily, monthly, quarterly, and half yearly goals, and look at each one and figure out what metric applies to each of them.

JAY'S GOAL TRACKING

I'll use my example from earlier and I'll break that down to show you how I would track each goal.

Daily Goal: Morning routine and workout
To track this, I would set up a spreadsheet calendar and I'd mark off each time I do my morning routine and workout.

Weekly Goal: Work out five times a week and keep within a five-pound weight range
To track workouts, I would use the calendar again. For keeping myself within my weight range, I'd weigh myself three times a week – on Sunday night to get an idea of where my week is starting, Wednesday night to check whether I've lost any pounds I might have gained over the weekend, and then again Friday morning to go into the weekend feeling good (as this is when I should be at my lowest weight).

This makes my Friday pizza night that much more guilt free. And on the flip side, if I had a bad eating week because I went out a bunch of times, and I weigh myself Friday morning and I'm up a few pounds, then I might not eat as many slices of pizza, or I'll fast for half a day on Saturday.

See how I'm tracking my weight with purpose to control my eating habits? I'm not just weighing myself every day and focusing on the number on the scale for no reason.

Monthly Goal: Lose one per cent body fat
Obviously for this goal, I'm going to measure my body fat at the start of the month and at the end of the month. BFP is a metric that takes a while to change. It's not something you measure all the time, like standing on a scale, so I wouldn't measure it any more than once a month. Generally, I like to measure it every six months, but I'm using the example of measuring once a month to show how it aligns with my monthly goal.

Quarterly Goal: Compete in a fitness competition
Competing in a fitness competition requires several factors to be exactly on point, all at the same time, to achieve that killer body you need to step on stage. You're tracking your workouts, your food, even how your body looks. I would need to track how many calories I was eating every day. I would even be tracking how much protein, fat and carbs I was eating. I would be taking progress photos every few weeks, so I could see what my body looked like, and I would be tracking BFP once a week as the competition date drew nearer. In short, I'd take this goal and break it up into all the things I need to track to ensure I achieve the best result possible.

Half Yearly Goal: Run a half marathon
For this goal, I wouldn't be tracking things like my BFP or my weight. I would be tracking how many kilometres I could run and, if I was trying to be competitive, how long it would take me to run them. Can you see how measuring anything else would be pointless?

Yearly Goal: Be in better shape than last year
This goal is kind of hard to track, isn't it? In light of this, I wouldn't be tracking this goal in any particular detail. Instead, I would say that if I completed all my other goals for the year, then I'd be in better shape than I was the previous year. Given this, my focus should be on completing those other goals, and tracking them to the best of my ability. That way, I can achieve them and, by extension, achieve my yearly goal.

TOOLS TO HELP MEASURE AND TRACK PROGRESS

I thought it might be useful to give you several tools that you can use to help measure yourself and track your progress. Some of them are pretty obvious and don't need much explaining, like a scale and a tape measure, but getting your BFP measured is a bit more complicated. I've compiled a list, which will help steer you in the right direction when you're ready to start tracking your progress.

Bathroom Scale
You're going to need a scale even if you aren't going to specifically track your weight, because, depending on which tool you use, you will need to know your weight in order to track your BFP.

I'm not going to recommend a specific one, as a scale is a scale. However, make sure that you use the same scale each time you weigh yourself. There is nothing more frustrating than realizing that the scale at the gym is off by three pounds compared to the one at home.

You can also buy scales that will measure BFP as well. A lot of them aren't particularly accurate, so I suggest doing some research to find out which ones are currently highly rated. You could use one to give yourself a benchmark to work off and, as long as you used the same one each time, you would be able to track your progress according to that number. It's a great option if you're just starting out and want to start measuring yourself.

Tape Measure

You will need a tape measure to take your body measurements. I like to use a tailor's soft tape measure because that's what it's designed for. Again, it's a pretty straightforward tool – you can pick one up online very easily. I suggest getting someone to help you with the measurements as it's hard to accurately measure yourself. Make sure that you take the measurements from the exact same spots when you redo them. I use markers like the belly button or the top of the hip bone to make sure I hit the same points every time.

BFP Scanner

When it comes to measuring BFP, there are a couple of options. One of my favourite choices, which I use for my clients, is the BodyMetrix™ Ultrasound System. This is very accurate, as it measures fat density at multiple sites across the body using an ultrasound wave that is administered through a non-invasive wand. The scanner plugs into a laptop and gives the user a detailed report on their BFP, water levels, fat thickness, and a few other points of reference.

Now, the unfortunate news is that these scanners are about $2,500, so it's probably not something you can afford to have sitting around your house. You might be able to find a health professional in your area who uses one, and who can administer a scan for you. If that's not possible, you can easily find someone to figure out your BFP with calipers, which I will discuss next.

BFP Calipers

Calipers measure subcutaneous fat, or fat located directly under your skin, by lightly pinching fat folds at different body sites. The data from the calipers, including information like your weight, height and age, is put into an equation, which will calculate your BFP. If done correctly, it will predict your BFP within three and a half per cent.

You can do this test yourself if you want to, but it needs to be done extremely accurately to get a proper calculation. I read somewhere that it takes about 200 attempts to get an accurate reading, so I suggest getting a fitness professional to administer the test. If possible, use the same person to conduct the test each time, so that it will be more accurate.

Spreadsheets, Calendars and Lists

A spreadsheet is a great tool to track all sorts of metrics. I like to print them off so that I can physically mark them. Create a workout spreadsheet or calendar, which you can mark off each day you do a workout. Create a list of the daily habits you want to achieve, so that you can mark them off as you do them. Create a calendar with your goals written on it, so that you can see what you are working toward this week, this month, and this year.

Don't underestimate these tools. Remember, the more you track your progress, the more likely you are to achieve your goals. I use physical calendars, printed spreadsheets, lists on my phone, computer, and pieces of paper all the time. This may sound childish, but you would be surprised how much easier it is to commit to something if you get to put a gold star sticker on a physical spreadsheet with your list of daily goals on it. Sometimes, all it takes is the act of ticking something off to help you stay on track.

Smart Fitness Trackers

At some point, you are going to need some sort of way to track how many calories you're burning throughout the day, so you can match that to your calorie intake. I'll be going into the finer details of this concept in chapter six, where I discuss nutrition in depth.

There's a variety of different companies that offer these kinds of trackers. Based on my research, they are all pretty much the same in terms of how they work, although some are tailored for specific purposes. It really depends on exactly what you want to use the tracker for. For example, if you only want to track calorie burn, then you can get something small and simple. Or if you want to track your sleep, and have other options like built-in music apps and phone call abilities, then you could get something like an Apple Watch or a Fitbit.

I currently use a Fitbit Ionic, which is the size of a watch. The reason I picked it is because, at the time, it was the only Fitbit that was waterproof. Some of the other trackers that interest me at the moment are the Oura Ring, which, as the name indicates, is a ring. I like this idea, as I'm not really a watch-wearing person.

Whoop bands are also gaining popularly. They come with a subscription service that you have to pay for, but you get access to a wide range of different metrics. If you're someone who loves numbers and wants to be tracking as much as possible, this could be a good option for you.

Accountability Partner

An accountability partner is one of the most underrated tools you can use to help keep you on track. Getting a work colleague or a friend involved in your journey is a great way to keep you motivated and accountable. It gives them an opportunity to improve their life as well, and have *you* as *their* support person. It can be as simple as going to the gym together, or even just regularly checking in on each other's progress. Not feeling like you're doing all this alone can serve as real encouragement and a great source of motivation to keep going.

CHAPTER SUMMARY

Remember, if you can't measure it, you can't improve it. Let me rephrase that as a question: If you don't measure it, how are you going to know you improved? Take measurements and track your results so that you know for sure that you are on the right path to achieving your health and fitness goals.

There are a lot of different ways to measure results, so make sure that you are using the right metrics for the right goal. If your goal is to lose fat but not weight, then weighing yourself every day isn't helpful. Recording your BFP is.

And most importantly, measuring your results and seeing your improvements is one of the best ways to boost your motivation and pump you up to continue focusing on your goals. You've worked hard. Wouldn't it make sense to have some tangible results you could see as a reward for your effort?

5

DISCIPLINE

You've now reached the third step in the Personal Revolution process: 'Discipline'. I'll be frank. At present, I believe this is the one major thing that sets me apart from you. I'm not smarter than you; there is no way I could do your job. I don't have more hours in my day than you do. I don't enjoy prepping food on Sundays, working out five days a week, or getting up early. Trust me – I don't. But I'm determined to achieve my goals, which requires a huge amount of discipline.

In fact, discipline could be the most important quality you need to have continued success long after the 'honeymoon' phase of your Personal Revolution is over. In this chapter, I'll explain why discipline is such a crucial part of your journey – and outline some proven ways to help you become more disciplined.

DISCIPLINE EQUALS FREEDOM

Discipline is defined as: 'To train oneself to do something in a controlled and habitual way.' Notice the use of the word 'habitual'? This is another word for 'habits'. Wouldn't you agree that most of the things you need to be doing to live a healthy life are really just good habits? Working out regularly, eating good food, getting a good night's sleep – these are all good habits.

But good habits don't just happen. They require you to be disciplined in order for them to become habits. For example, in order for me to write this book, I used my discipline to get up at 4:00 a.m. Monday to Friday to write for an hour. I don't normally get up at 4:00 a.m. (this isn't a normal habit), so it was pure discipline that got me out of bed for those first few days, even when every part of me was telling me to stay in bed.

A couple of times, I came close to turning my alarm off and going back to sleep. However, after a week or two of this practice, I noticed that getting up wasn't necessarily getting easier – it's not like I wanted to get up at 4:00 a.m. – but it was becoming a habit and didn't require as much discipline. I wasn't battling myself like I was in the first week.

There is a great concept and phrase: *'Discipline Equals Freedom'*. There is a great book by the same name written by Jocko Willink, a former Navy SEAL commander.

> *'If you don't think you are disciplined: It is because you haven't decided to be disciplined. YET.'*
> – JOCKO WILLINK

I think it's easier if I just give you some examples of how discipline equals freedom, so you can understand how this concept applies to your Personal Revolution:

If every Sunday I was disciplined and cooked five lunches for my work week, I'd have the freedom to not worry about lunch every workday, and I'd save time in my evenings by not having to prepare meals.

- If I was disciplined and created a workout plan for every day of the week, I'd have the freedom to not dwell on the type of workout I should do each day, or if I'm even going to work out. Instead, I'd just have to follow the plan.
- If I was disciplined from Sunday to Friday and never overate, I would have the freedom to eat whatever I wanted on Saturday.
- If, every pay day, I was disciplined enough to put ten per cent of my pay into a holiday fund, at the end of the year I would have the freedom to book a holiday anywhere in the world.
- If I was disciplined and packed my bag the night before, and put my clothes out for the next day, I would have the freedom to create a less hectic morning routine because I wouldn't be so focused on trying to prepare for work.

You can see from these examples that by being disciplined and creating these habits, you've suddenly freed up time to focus on other things and you've made these positive changes a lot easier to stick to.

THE LINK BETWEEN DISCIPLINE AND HABITS

Now that I've mentioned the word 'habits', I want to explain the link between discipline and habits, so that you understand how to make proper use of each to your advantage. Remember, as I said earlier, discipline could be the major difference between you and me, so I don't want you reading through this chapter without really understanding why this is so important and how you can become more disciplined in your personal life.

Remember in chapter three when I said goals and motivation are a bit like the chicken and the egg? Well, discipline and habits are the same, in that it's hard to know which comes first. You need discipline to create a habit, but you need a habit in order to exercise discipline.

I believe that you need to be cultivating them both at the same time, yet thinking about them as two separate skill sets. You need to recognize them both as you're trying to incorporate them into your life. That way, you can see yourself not only creating good habits, but becoming more disciplined, which will encourage you to maintain your good habits.

You need to create a conscious feedback loop that gets stronger and stronger the longer you stay in it. Let's say, for example, you want to work out every day Monday through Friday. For this to become a habit, you decide, 'I'm going to get up at 6:00 a.m. each day so I can go to the gym. This is my new habit.'

The first week, you get up at 6:00 a.m. every day and you make it to the gym. This isn't a habit yet; you're just using motivation to get yourself out of bed. You think this is a new habit because you're feeling motivated and you're actually getting up, but it's not. Second week comes along, you get up on Monday at 6:00 a.m., Tuesday at 6:00 a.m., but then you work late and you don't sleep well Tuesday night.

The alarm goes off Wednesday at 6:00 a.m. and suddenly you're at the critical flashpoint for this good habit that is beginning to form. Motivation is now gone, so are you going to use discipline and get up still, or hit snooze and skip the gym? If you don't use discipline, this new routine, which could have become a habit, is now gone. If you hit snooze, chances of you getting up on Thursday at 6:00 a.m. are now minimal, and the chances of forming this habit (of getting up at 6:00 a.m. to work out) are nonexistent.

Had you said to yourself, 'No, I need to be disciplined in order for this to become my new habit,' you would have got up and done your workout. You would have been tired, but you would have felt so accomplished and proud of yourself for being self-disciplined. Guess what? Now you're motivated again, and you get up for the rest of the week, no problem. You're creating this never-ending feedback loop, turning your routine into a habit, and making the habit stronger and stronger the longer you maintain it.

For the remainder of this chapter, I'll share with you my top tips for becoming more disciplined.

CREATE A MORNING ROUTINE

'In the right hands, [a routine] can be a finely calibrated mechanism for taking advantage of a range of limited resources: time (the most limited resource of all) as well as willpower, self-discipline, optimism. A solid routine fosters a well-worn groove for one's mental energies and helps stave off the tyranny of moods.'
– MASON CURREY, AUTHOR OF *DAILY RITUALS: HOW ARTISTS WORK*

For you to become more disciplined, I'm going to suggest that you start with a proper morning routine. Now, a proper morning routine doesn't mean you get up as late as you can before work, rush around deciding what you're going to wear for the day, start looking at your emails and social media, drink a coffee as you run out the door, and perhaps even take a phone call. A proper morning routine is a specific, planned, conscious routine that allows you to 'boot up' or start your day exactly the same way each day, in control and with a purpose. If you want to be more disciplined, then you need to make the first minutes of your day an act of self-discipline. If you want to feel in control of your personal life, then it's important to take control from the moment you wake up.

As Tim Ferriss, entrepreneur and bestselling author says, '*If you win the morning, you win the day.*' Studies have shown that having a routine can reduce stress, improve your health, and even create a more meaningful life. By creating a morning routine and completing it each day, you've accomplished something important to you as the first task of the day.

Once you do create a morning routine, imagine how you're going to feel walking out the door to go to work. You're going to have a sense of pride, and are more likely going to tick something else off your list of things you want to do for the day. If eating healthy and getting to the gym is on that list, chances are you're going to complete those tasks as well. When you do something positive, you feel happier and you feel motivated. Something triggers your brain to want to do something else positive. It's a snowball effect that you could trigger immediately every day. Personally, I want to feel motivated and good about myself from the moment I walk outside – not stressed, running late, and feeling like everything is in chaos already.

When it comes to creating your morning routine, have some fun with it; it doesn't need to be stressful. *Don't* overthink it. One of the biggest mistakes my clients make is they create these elaborate morning routines, which sound amazing on paper but end up taking too much time and effort and are never completed properly. Remember, the point is that you are trying to create a routine that you can 100 per cent complete every morning, so that you feel good about yourself and can use that positivity for the rest of your day. If you're never *quite* completing your morning routine, then you're going to be frustrated, which is the opposite effect of what you want.

Your morning routine should be unique to you, it should be something that you create on your own, and something that you want to do. I'm going to give you some guidelines that I think are important to follow, but, ultimately, it's up to you. I'll even share my current morning routine with you, so that you can see what I do. Feel free to grab some ideas for yourself, but what I do might not be the best routine for you. We are all unique and what works for me might do the opposite for you.

Your morning routine might take you only two minutes, five minutes, fifteen minutes, or could even be as long as sixty minutes. It can be extremely detailed, minute by minute, or can be relaxed and flowing. As long as you can easily complete it every day without fail, it doesn't matter. As long as you're ticking off something within each of these four categories, you can set it up however you like:

- Health
- Mindfulness
- Movement
- Written

Health

Health means doing something that is good for your health, such as brushing your teeth, drinking a glass of lemon-infused water, and taking your multivitamin. You want to be consciously doing something that is healthy as soon as you start your day. This way, you're more likely to tick other healthy things off your list during the day.

Mindfulness

Mindfulness means doing something that is good for your mind, such as some form of meditation, breathing exercises, listening to a mindfulness podcast, or taking a walk without your phone. It's important to give yourself the mental space to think about what you're doing for the day, or your life's bigger picture. Better yet, try to spend some time not thinking of anything at all.

Movement

Movement means doing something that gets your body moving, such as a ten-minute stretch routine, going for a walk, doing twenty push-ups – anything to get your body moving. You've been lying down in bed for hopefully at least six hours, so you want to get your blood flowing and wake up your body – particularly since you likely sit at a desk all day. If this is the case, all you're doing is going from lying down to sitting down for hours on end, so it's no wonder your body isn't looking and feeling its best.

Written

Written means doing something that requires you to go through the act of writing something down, be it a five-minute journaling exercise, a checklist for the day, or something you're grateful for. It's important to give yourself a moment to think and write. Your head is no doubt constantly swirling with different thoughts, but there is something very therapeutic about putting pen to paper. And yes, I do recommend using a pen and paper rather than typing. You will find there is something very tangible and real to writing on paper, which is different from typing on a phone or computer.

Interested to see what a morning routine might look like? Here's mine...

JAY'S MORNING ROUTINE

I get up exactly one hour before I start work.

I check my phone for any overnight client cancellation messages, but nothing else. I want to be phone free for the first thirty minutes of my day. (Mindfulness)

I go to the bathroom.

I weigh myself, just to keep a check on what my body is doing. (Health)

I drink as much water as I can. (Health)

I get dressed.

I do a series of movements: ten arm swings, ten squats, as many push-ups as I can, ten toe touches, ten glute activations, and ten leg swings. (Movement)

I sit in a specific chair and do a ten-minute guided meditation through an app. (Mindfulness)

I turn on my coffee machine and prepare a coffee.

I write down three different things I'm grateful for and I put them into a jar. Google 'gratitude jar' if you want to see the concept behind it. (Written, Mindfulness)

I sit down at the kitchen counter with my coffee and I spend five minutes writing in my journal. I write down two things I want to achieve for the day, a checklist for anything I need to do that day, and, finally, any thoughts, ideas or musings I may have. (Written)

I pick up my phone and reply to any overnight texts from family and friends who are overseas, check and delete my emails from overnight, and play games on my iPad.

Finally, I brush my teeth. (Health)

CREATE AN EVENING ROUTINE

It's a well-known fact that most of the highly successful people in the world have some sort of morning routine. You can find all sorts of podcasts and books on the topic of morning routines. Google 'morning routine' and you will come across enough content on the topic to dive as deep as you want into it. However, there isn't as much of a discussion around evening routines.

I think creating an evening routine is highly underrated, and I think it's crucial for anyone who is overworked, tired and trying to create some structure around their life outside of work. Particularly for people working long hours, in high-pressure jobs, there comes a point in every day when you have to get out of your own head, switch off, and transfer all your mental energy toward making conscious, positive decisions that are only about what's best for you – not what you need to get done.

Think about your current day-to-day life. It's probably chaos from the moment you get up, as you deal with emails, calls, texts, meetings, pitches, presentations, events and deadlines. Let's say you incorporate a morning routine just like I suggest. However, that doesn't stop the emails, calls, texts and so on that come with the nature of your position. So if you let all that noise follow you right up to the moment you try to fall asleep, I'm almost willing to bet that you don't sleep well, and you don't sleep for at least seven hours a night.

Ninety-nine per cent of all the executives I've worked with over the years are in this situation, so that's why I'm pretty confident you are as well. An evening routine creates an 'off' switch. More than that, it creates some personal time, dedicated only to you, which you give to yourself.

I don't care how much you get paid; your company doesn't own every second you have until the moment you close your eyes at night. Remember, the whole reason why most people aren't successfully managing a career, and experiencing a level of personal health and physical appearance they are happy with, is because they haven't taken ownership of their personal time. In fact, they don't *have* any time; they have given it all away.

Your evening routine is going to take some of that time back. I want you to think about your evening routine as your shutdown sequence, just like the morning routine was your boot-up. Same as the morning routine, it doesn't have to be a specific amount of time – it could be fifteen minutes, or it could be an hour. Ideally, I would suggest the longer you can give yourself the better, but start off small. Again, it has to be something you can commit to without fail. You're trying to build discipline, so you don't want it to be so elaborate that every second or third evening you end up not doing it. That defeats the point.

Unlike your morning routine, I don't have specific categories that I think should be included. However, I do have a lot of suggestions and, again, I'll share with you my evening routine, which you're welcome to take inspiration from. The morning routine is very specific, as it's designed to put your body and mind into an optimized state before you walk out the door. When it comes to the evening routine, I want you to get out of your head, take back some of your own time, and be deliberate and purposeful with yourself, so that you can go to bed feeling like you're in the driver's seat of your life.

10 Tips to Create an Effective Evening Routine

Here is a list of some points and suggestions I have around figuring out your evening routine:

1. At some point in the evening, you have to stop working. You need to make a conscious decision to say, 'That's it'. That has to be the starting point to your brain switching off. Part of this could be putting your phone away – that's a great way to start your evening routine.
2. Evening routines are a great time to take any supplements or focus on any specific health regimens you want to be following. You don't forget if it becomes part of the routine.
3. Try to stop looking at screens at least thirty minutes before bed. Before you roll your eyes at that, consider this: studies show that the blue light coming from electronic devices stops your body from producing melatonin, a hormone you need to go to sleep.
4. Read a book. There is no better way to distract yourself from today's or tomorrow's stress than reading.
5. Shower, brush your teeth, and moisturize your face. You probably do these things already, but you can still include them in your routine, as they're all part of the shutdown sequence.
6. Write a to-do list for the following day, so you aren't lying in bed thinking about what you need to do tomorrow. Having it written down means you aren't going to forget and it's out of mind.
7. Journal. Spend five minutes writing down your thoughts on the day, plus two good things that happened, or why tomorrow is going to be a good day. If you don't know where to start, just buy a pre-structured journal and fill in the prompts. Don't overthink it – any kind of journaling is better than nothing.
8. Do a stretch sequence, a five-minute yoga routine, or something similar to help you relax and wind down.
9. Prepare your lunch for the next day.
10. Put your clothes out for the next day. If you're planning on

going to the gym in the morning, then packing your gym bag is an important part of your evening routine to help ensure you get up and go.

This is a great list of ideas and starting points for your new evening routine. Remember to start off small, as you can always add to it once it has become an automatic habit. Here is my current evening routine as of writing. You're welcome to add any parts of it to your own routine if you think they make sense for you.

JAY'S EVENING ROUTINE

I put on my blue light blocking glasses around 7:00 p.m.

I check my schedule for the following day, making sure I reply to any unanswered texts. I then put my phone on charge, meaning no more social media, emails, and so on from around 8:00 p.m.

I take my evening supplements.

I take a shower.

I do my skincare regimen.

I brush my teeth.

I take my journal and iPad into my room.

I fill out my journal. I'm currently using *The Freedom Journal* by John Lee Dumas. This simple journal gets me to highlight the positives and negatives from my day, what I need to be grateful for, and what I want out of tomorrow. It takes two minutes to fill out, which I like.

During whatever time I have left between then and 9:30 p.m., I read a book on my iPad.

I set an alarm for the morning.

I take off my blue light blocking glasses and, if possible, turn the light off no later than 9:30 p.m.

FOUR OTHER WAYS TO BECOME MORE DISCIPLINED

Now that we've spent some time talking about becoming more disciplined through morning and evening routines, I hope you're starting to see how vital discipline is to becoming that fit, healthy person you've always wanted to be. Like I said at the start of this chapter, one of the major differences between you and me is discipline. So I want to give you as many tools as possible for you to become more disciplined, so that when you move into the next section of the book, where you learn about nutrition and working out, you won't fail at integrating these changes permanently.

Here are a few things for you to think about and take on board.

Acknowledge Your Weaknesses
We all have weaknesses. It's normal. For most successful, career-driven people, the idea of acknowledging any weaknesses is extremely hard. If you've been crushing it in your career for many

years, I'm guessing you didn't get there by being vulnerable and admitting when you were doing something wrong. That just makes you driven, not disciplined.

Understanding where your weaknesses are, once you step out of the office, is a key component to dealing with them. For example, if you drink six coffees a day but refuse to acknowledge it's a problem, then what are the chances that you're going to reduce that number? Similarly, we all know a smoker who never admits that smoking is bad for them. These people are far less likely to stop smoking, simply because they refuse to acknowledge how unhealthy it is.

Acknowledge your flaws; don't pretend they don't exist. Once you admit to them, you can change them. I think one of the reasons clients love working with me so much is because I will call them out when they act like what they are doing isn't bad for them. Some require more work than others, and this comes down to your attitude. I can give you all the best workouts and nutrition tips in the world, but if you don't acknowledge your weak points and try to fix them, it's nearly pointless trying to implement those other changes.

Remove Temptations

This one is kind of obvious, but it's worth reminding you. If you're trying to eat better at home and you have junk food in your pantry, get rid of it. One of the very first things I do with someone who has signed up for my Personal Revolution intensive program is go to their house with a garbage bag and remove any junk food and other unhealthy items from their fridge and cupboards. I've literally filled bag loads of stuff that needs to be thrown out.

If you're serious about winning your Personal Revolution, you need to remove temptations as much as you can. Using the earlier example of drinking too much coffee, if you have a serious coffee addiction then you might have to get rid of your coffee machine. A Personal Revolution is an all or nothing cause. In order to win, you must be willing to do whatever it takes.

Understand There is Never a 'Right Time'

If you want to become more disciplined, and, as a result, change your life, start now. There is no perfect time. There is no point reading this book and deciding you'll implement these changes in a few months when things at work aren't as busy. When is your workplace ever not busy?

The first step toward becoming disciplined is doing that first thing you don't want to do. If you don't start this journey now, the chances of starting later are slim to none. I can say this to you with conviction because, over the years, I've had hundreds of people ask me about coaching programs, personal training or joining my boot camp classes. I've heard plenty of people say things like, 'I think I'll join when the weather is nicer', 'I'm not quite ready', 'I'll join the next program', 'I'll join when I'm not so busy', and 'I'll sign up when I lose a few pounds on my own first'. Among those people, I'd say more than ninety per cent never join up at a later date.

The ones who *are* serious try the free class as soon as possible, sign up for a consultation straightaway, typically stay on and end up achieving their goals, and, ultimately, are successful in changing their life. So, the key is to get started *now*, and it all starts by taking that first step.

Don't Always Pick the Path of Least Resistance

As Theodore Roosevelt said, '*With great victory comes great sacrifice.*' You need to push yourself a little if you're going to build self-discipline. I don't expect you to sacrifice everything in order to achieve excellence in your Personal Revolution. However, considering you have already sacrificed your health and fitness up to this point in your life, I want you to put a bit of that hard grit you've put into your career into your personal life. If it's too easy, you aren't going to reach your full potential.

I understand this is a fine line. Earlier, I said I don't want you to push yourself to 100 per cent. Otherwise, you're going to burn out and give up. However, I also don't want you to *not* push yourself hard enough. If you're going to put the effort into this, I don't want you to waste your opportunity to grow as much as you can, or miss out on that deep level of satisfaction that comes from digging deep and achieving something you had to work hard for.

For example, I got up at 4:00 a.m. Monday to Friday in order to write this book within eight weeks. I normally get up at 5:15 a.m., so 4:00 a.m. wasn't way out of my comfort zone but it was challenging for me, no doubt about it. But it gave me a real sense of pride that I was able to push myself this way. Realistically, I probably could have found time to write this book in the afternoons, but that was the path of least resistance and I wanted the opportunity to grow as a person while I wrote this book. Getting up at 4:00 a.m. day after day requires an incredible amount of discipline, so I'm proud of myself for doing it.

CHAPTER SUMMARY

By implementing a morning routine, an evening routine, and the four other tactics I shared to become more disciplined, I hope you can see yourself as more likely to succeed in your Personal Revolution. It's not easy. Otherwise everyone would be doing it. But with the right tools, and an understanding of the fundamentals on how to prepare yourself, you can now move into the final section of this book, which is all about fighting to win your Personal Revolution.

6

NUTRITION

Now you reach the fourth step in the Personal Revolution process: 'Nutrition'. Please note that I am not a registered nutritionist or dietitian, so I'm not going to give you specific advice on exactly which foods or supplements you should be taking. What I *am* going to do is share what works for me personally. I'm also going to explore some different topics and principles involving nutrition and dieting, and what's happening inside your body, so that you can understand how it all goes together. Hopefully then you will see why it's so important to pay attention to what and how much you eat, and to eat with purpose and clarity.

I think it is very important for everyone to understand how their body works, particularly when it comes to nutrition. After all, it's what keeps your body going, and determines whether or not you feel good, are physically and mentally healthy, lose weight or gain muscle, and so on. It's the foundation of staying alive, yet most people have no idea how it all works. Therefore, I encourage you to educate yourself further on this topic. However, if you can get a firm grasp of everything in this chapter, and diligently apply these principles, you will be able to look after yourself for the rest of your life.

ARE YOU SETTING YOURSELF UP TO FAIL?

Before I break down how your metabolism, calories and diets work, let's go through some common ways you might be setting yourself up to fail. That way, you can nip anything in the bud before it becomes too problematic. Nutrition (what you eat) is the number one factor in determining what your body looks like. If you want to change how your body looks, the first thing you need to look at is your nutritional intake. With that in mind, here are four common mistakes people make when it comes to nutrition.

Overcomplicating It

One of the big mistakes people make with nutrition is that they overcomplicate it. When something becomes very complicated, it becomes harder and harder to maintain. You have to remind yourself: 'Where on the scale of zero to 100 am I trying to sit, and are my diet and nutrition choices matching that position?'

When I competed in a natural bodybuilding show, I was counting out exact grams of protein and carbs in every single meal for months at a time. Think about the amount of time I spent focusing on my diet, weighing and calculating everything. I was trying to sit at 100 per cent on that scale to compete in that show, whereas I don't do that now at all.

Worrying about the exact timing of when you eat protein versus fat and carbs, and exactly how many grams of each you're eating, is pointless if you don't even know how many calories you're burning or eating in a day. I could write a whole book on nutrition, but the point of a Personal Revolution is to create change in your life that is permanent, and to have balance between your career and time spent on yourself. Don't overcomplicate your eating habits and nutrition. Instead, figure out what twenty per cent of changes will make eighty per cent of the improvements, and focus on that for now. Make it simple so you can follow the guidelines and get the results you want.

Being Too Extreme or Strict

Another reason people set themselves up to fail is being too extreme or strict about their diet, and this goes hand in hand with overcomplicating it. If you make your diet too extreme and strict all at once, the likelihood of you staying on it is slim.

Changing your diet drastically can also cause your body to go into a state of near shock. If you don't believe me, try giving up sugar and coffee completely for the next few days, and tell me how you feel! Feelings of withdrawal are not uncommon. In fact, mood swings, headaches, mental and physical fatigue, overemotional outbursts and irritability are just some of the potential signs of a diet being too extreme. No one should be feeling this way.

On the contrary, making changes to your diet should give you a clearer head, make you feel happier, and give you more energy. This circles back to the eighty per cent rule. Often, when someone goes on a diet, it's at 100 per cent, which is an unrealistic expectation to put on yourself.

I've repeatedly watched people go from eating whatever they want to cutting sugar, caffeine, carbs and dairy, and the number of calories they are consuming, all at once. Imagine how you would feel trying to do that for the next seven days. Maybe you've even tried that in the past. If so, how long did you last? I'm going to guess it wasn't very long, and, if you did manage to last six weeks or so, what happened when you stopped? Did you go back to exactly the same habits as before?

Don't be too strict on yourself. Remember, your Personal Revolution is a change you're making for life, not a quick eight-week fix to lose as much weight as possible.

Having the Wrong Mindset

Having the wrong mindset is another key reason people end up abandoning healthier eating habits. Thinking that you are on a 'diet' now is a sure way of eventually giving up and reverting back to 'normal' eating. This time, you need to focus on the ways in which healthier eating aligns with your goals and your vision for yourself.

That doesn't mean that, from now on, you're always on a diet. It's always your choice. There is nothing worse than treating yourself like a bad child and going through life depriving yourself of opportunities because you're 'on a diet' and you're 'not allowed'. I see this all the time. In fact, it's probably one of the most common mistakes I see people making. They're constantly in conflict with themselves over what they can and can't eat.

My goal with this chapter is to educate you with enough knowledge so that you can get an understanding of how your body works and how to eat with purpose to match your goals. Personally, I never miss an opportunity to eat something I really want. I just have a better understanding of the cause and effect of those choices, so I make them with my head up, owning the outcomes.

Lacking the Right Knowledge

That brings me to the last major reason people set themselves up to fail. Quite simply, they don't have the knowledge. Nutrition is complicated; studying it can require an entire university degree. It's not surprising, then, that most people have no understanding about calories, how their metabolism works, or how the foods they are eating are truly affecting their body and their health.

How can you expect to eat well and look after yourself if you really have no idea what's going on? Simply following whatever the new catchphrase diet is, without understanding the science behind it, is stupid in my opinion. If you don't know what that diet is or isn't supposed to do, then you're going into it completely blind and it could possibly end up having the opposite effect from what you want.

Take the time to educate yourself enough so that you feel in control of your situation. It's exactly the same as in your profession. If you have people or other departments that report to you, you need to have some knowledge of what their roles are. You don't need to be an expert, but, if you have no idea what they are talking about, then how do you know if they are doing a good job or not? Similarly, you don't need to become a nutritionist to look after yourself, but you do need to have a basic understanding of what's going on.

Now that you're aware of some of the common mistakes that may be delaying your journey to healthier eating and better nutritional habits, let's start looking into how all this stuff actually works in a way that is easy to understand and apply.

UNDERSTANDING YOUR METABOLISM

'Metabolism'. What does this word even mean? I'm sure you've heard people say things like, 'I can't lose weight; I have a very slow metabolism.' Or, on the flip side, 'I can eat anything; I have a fast metabolism.' The definition of 'metabolism', according to the *Encyclopedia Britannica*, is: 'The sum of the chemical reactions that take place within each cell of a living organism and that provide energy for vital processes and for synthesizing new organic material.' How's that for scientific jargon?!

How about this? Your metabolism refers to the breakdown of food being converted to energy. That's already easier to understand. Your metabolism isn't just one thing. It's a whole process of storing energy, converting food to fuel for energy, and burning that fuel for energy. In layman's terms, when people refer to their metabolism, they are really referring to the amount of food or calories they can eat each day without gaining or losing weight.

There are a few components to your metabolism, which I think are important for us to cover so that you have a better understanding of how your body works. I find that with most clients, once they understand the relationship between the food they eat and their body, it puts the ownership of looking after their body and health back into their hands.

Basal Metabolic Rate
Basal Metabolic Rate (BMR) is the amount of energy or calories required to keep you alive. Surprisingly, you actually burn through a lot of calories just living. Imagine you lay in bed all day without

moving – just your heart beating and your lungs breathing. That's what your BMR calorie amount is.

Interestingly, your BMR accounts for sixty to eighty per cent of your total daily energy expenditure, or the number of calories you need to eat every day. So, if you're trying to figure out how much food you should be eating each day, you can see that it's probably pretty important to have a rough idea what your BMR is. I personally would recommend getting some sort of fitness tracker, which can track your entire day's calorie expenditure.

Alternatively, you can use the Harris-Benedict formula, which takes into consideration your weight, height and age to give you an estimate of your BMR. Here are some examples:

Men: BMR = 66 + (6.2 × weight in pounds) + (12.7 × height in inches) − (6.76 × age in years)

Women: BMR = 655 + (4.35 × weight in pounds) + (4.7 × height in inches) − (4.7 × age in years)

This calculation looks quite confusing, doesn't it? So let me show you how to use it using myself as an example. The easiest way to do this is first calculate the numbers that are in the brackets and then add or subtract them.

Jay's BMR

1. 6.2 x **170 pounds** (my weight) = 1,054
2. 12.7 x **70 inches** (my height) = 889
3. 6.76 x **37 years** (my age) = 250

66 + 1,054 + 889 − 250 = 1,759 calories

Looking at this number, I now know that I need to eat at least 1,759 calories a day to give my body what it needs to survive.

Total Daily Energy Expenditure

Once you have figured out what your BMR is, then the next thing you can estimate is your total daily energy expenditure (TDEE), which is the total amount of energy or calories you burn every day.

Now, this number will change every day depending on what you're doing. For example, if you spend a whole day running around doing chores and then a workout, your TDEE is going to be a lot higher than if you spend a lazy Sunday on the couch watching Netflix.

So, once you've estimated your BMR using the Harris-Benedict formula, your next step to figuring out your TDEE is to include the number of calories you burn during daily activities based on your lifestyle:

- **Sedentary:** If you get minimal or no exercise, multiply your BMR by 1.2.
- **Lightly active:** If you exercise lightly one to three days a week, multiply your BMR by 1.375.
- **Moderately active:** If you exercise moderately three to five days a week, multiply your BMR by 1.55.
- **Very active:** If you engage in intense exercise six to seven days a week, multiply your BMR by 1.725.
- **Extra active:** If you engage in very intense exercise six to seven days a week or have a physically demanding job, multiply your BMR by 1.9.

Remember this is only an estimate, but it will give you a very good idea of the minimum and maximum number of calories you should be consuming on a daily basis. I like to calculate both 'sedentary' and 'extra active' because we all have those days where we sit around doing nothing, and I want to know what my TDEE is going to be for days like that.

Jay's TDEE

Using my BMR from the calculation of 1,759 calories, I need to select from the list what sort of lifestyle I live. I fall under the **Extra Active** category, so I need to multiply my 1,759 by 1.9. Therefore, my TDEE is 3,342 calories. You can see now I need to be eating a lot of food to sustain myself every day. What about you? How much do you actually need?

If you know that on days you do nothing you only burn, let's say, 2,000 calories, and you decide that you're going to eat a full bag of chips and a pizza, then for sure you're going to overeat that day, calorie wise. On the flip side, if you have a really busy day and you've been super active, and you know that your TDEE is closer to 3,000 calories, then having an extra slice of pizza or some dessert isn't going to be the worst thing for you. In other words, you won't be overeating that day due to how active you've been.

Speeding Up Versus Slowing Down

The last point I want to cover about metabolism is this idea about speeding up or slowing down your metabolism. Yes, it is true that some people have a faster metabolism, and some have a slower one. This means that someone whose body has a fast metabolism burns more energy just to keep it running.

Going back to what the BMR refers to (the energy required to keep your body alive) one person might require 1,500 calories, while another person of the exact same weight and age might burn 2,000 calories. That means that without even doing anything, that first person can eat 500 calories more without it affecting their weight. They have a faster metabolism. The biggest determining factor for whether you have a fast or slow metabolism is genetics. Every organ in your body requires energy to run, and that person with the faster metabolism might just happen to have a bigger liver and heart, which require more energy to run.

No products out there can permanently speed up your metabolism, so forget about fat burners and other supplements that claim to do that. One of the only ways you can speed up your metabolism is to start heavy weight training with the purpose of building muscle. The more muscle you have, the more energy your body is going to need to run it. The other great aspect of weight training is that you actually burn calories while you are training, which means you need to eat more to sustain your workout. I love food, so, for me personally, I want to be burning as many calories as possible each day so I can eat more food without putting weight on.

CALORIES IN, CALORIES OUT

Let's talk about calories – a topic most people don't want to read about or learn about. It's complicated, so I'm going to give you just enough information to look after your body. Think of this as me teaching you basic math. I'm teaching you enough skills so that your level of math can get you through life. Yes, if you wanted to be an astrophysicist, your math skills would have to be way more advanced, but that's not what we are trying to achieve here. This level of nutritional understanding will keep you in control of your eating habits.

Now, before we go any further, I have to warn you. If you're like one of the many clients who have told me they will do anything to change their diet, but then refuse to count their calories, then I'm sorry – you're in for a rude awakening. Unless you can confidently tell me exactly how many calories you ate yesterday, or even just how many calories your breakfast contained today, then you're going to have to count your calories at some point if you truly want the body and physical fitness you aspire to.

I'm going to remind you again. Close to 100 per cent of what your body looks like comes down to the kind of food, and the amount of food, you're eating. Obviously, the muscle and tone of your body comes from working out. But if you have ten to twenty pounds of fat to lose, you aren't losing that on a treadmill. Without going into all the math, a rough estimate of time to lose one pound on a treadmill is six to ten hours. You can comfortably lose one to two pounds a week without working out at all, just by changing your eating habits. I know what I would rather do.

'Calories in, calories out' simply means that in order for your body to stay exactly the same weight, shape and size, it requires the exact same number of calories to be eaten (in) as the number of calories that were used during that day (out). If I had an active day and I burnt 3,000 calories for the entire day, and I ate 3,000 calories, I wouldn't gain or lose weight. Now, if I had a very lazy day and only burnt 2,000 calories, but I ate 3,000 calories worth of food, guess what happens to the extra 1,000 calories I just ate?

Some of that is going to turn to body fat. Imagine this happens on a daily basis. This is essentially how you put weight on over time.

COUNTING CALORIES

Now we get to the counting calories part. If you don't know exactly how many calories you're eating every day, then how do you know whether you're overeating every day? Unfortunately, the only way you are truly going to understand how much you are consuming, and how that compares to how much you're burning, is to count your calories.

What's really unfortunate in today's society is that, with all the processed food available, it's almost impossible to determine exactly how many calories a food item contains unless you read the label. Once you start doing this, you're going to be shocked. It doesn't matter if it's 'healthy' or not. Sometimes, a particular item of food can contain a huge number of calories – to the point that you might think, 'Surely it couldn't be that much.'

For example, one day I was at the shops, doing some chores, when I realized I was quite hungry. I grabbed a small pack of some sort of 'power' balls (the kind made up of nuts, dates, seeds, honey, and so on). There were about ten of these balls in the pack, each about an inch in diameter, so not big at all. For some reason, I didn't check the label to look at the calories, and I ended up eating the entire pack as I walked around. When I was done, I looked at the label and realized that each ball was eighty calories. That meant I had just eaten 800 calories as a snack while I walked around the shops. Why I remember this so vividly is because at the time I was dieting for a fitness show and I was only eating 1,800 calories a day. I had just eaten almost half the number of calories for my day in one snack. I couldn't believe it.

How often do you think you put yourself in this situation unwillingly? I thought to myself, 'I'm doing something good. I've made the smart choice. I picked out a healthy snack with no added sugars.' Yet I ate way more than I was anticipating. To avoid making this mistake, and derailing your health and fitness efforts, you need to start educating yourself about what you're eating. Notice I'm not telling you what you *should* eat. Instead, I'm telling you to gain a better understanding of the number of calories you're eating. Big difference.

Counting calories shouldn't be something you have to do for life, but it may be something you need to do for at least a month in order to cover all the different kinds of foods you eat, and to give yourself enough education on just how many calories are in the typical foods you eat.

Don't look at this as a negative experience. Rather, treat it as an opportunity to educate yourself. Once you know how many calories are in something, you can make a better-informed choice about whether you really want to eat it – and in what quantity and how often. It's very powerful because it means you're suddenly in the driver's seat of your dieting and nutrition. Personally, I don't want to be eating something, thinking that it's healthy, or low in calories, when in fact it isn't. If I'm going to eat half a pizza, I need to know that it contains 1,300 calories. And if I've eaten a lot of food already that day, then I know I'm overeating and potentially going to put weight on. Then it's my choice.

Now, unfortunately, that first month is going to be a real pain to figure out. How are you going to count the calories you consume at home if you prepare any meals for yourself? You're going to have to weigh food on a scale and calculate each individual ingredient of a recipe to ensure that you know the exact calories in a meal and a serving.

What if every day you're overeating? Don't you want to know that? If you knew that a certain salad dressing would increase the calories in your lunchtime salad from 300 to 600, would you reduce or remove the dressing altogether? What if you realized that your Starbucks grande latte contains 190 calories, whereas a black coffee with a splash of milk is only about twenty calories?

Trust me. If you take the time to educate yourself on your eating and drinking habits, you won't believe all the little places you're consuming unbelievable amounts of calories without even realizing it. Once you truly know how many calories you're consuming in a day, you're then able to start manipulating that to your advantage to lose or gain weight.

MEAL PREP 101

When it comes to controlling your calorie intake, obviously the easiest way to do this is by preparing your own meals at home. Or, as many people like to call it, meal prep. By preparing your meals at home, you have full control of exactly what goes into each meal and how it's made, which is important when you're trying to make sure you aren't overeating each day.

One way to do this is by simply ordering food via a healthy meal delivery service, which will deliver precooked meals to your home once or twice a week, depending on how many you order. Think of the time you could save at lunchtime or even at dinnertime if you had some pre-made meals in containers that you could heat up in the microwave or oven in five minutes.

Instead of spending thirty minutes of your lunch break walking back and forth to a shop, and waiting in a line for food, you could take back some of that time for yourself. Or in the evening, if you came home and there was some food waiting for you to eat, you might get back thirty minutes of your evening to relax instead of prepping and cooking food. The nice thing about ordering food through a meal delivery service is that you know exactly how many calories your meal contains without weighing or measuring anything.

I've had clients in the past who have ended up relying on meal delivery for almost all their meals for the week. They were happy to reheat a meal two or three times a day, and to eat a simpler diet. I'm not going to tell you that is wrong; if it works for you and you're happy with it, then go ahead. If that's what it takes for you to take control of your nutritional intake, then it's a great option. However, I suggest that a more hands-on approach to your meal prep is a better long-term option.

Remember, the whole point of having a Personal Revolution is for *you* to take control and ownership of your personal health and fitness, which means the more you do yourself, the more you're in charge. It's why I get all my personal training clients to work out on their own in between their sessions with me.

Anyone can meal prep on their own at home; I won't accept the excuse that you don't know how to cook. If you're intelligent enough to read this book, you're smart enough to be able to prepare five lunch meals a week. I'm going to give you two examples of how easy it is, step by step, so you have no excuse as to why you can't be doing this yourself.

The first example shows that you don't even need to cook anything. It's a salad.

PREPARING A SALAD

1. Go to a homewares store and buy five glass containers with lids.

2. Go to the grocery store, buy a bag of salad mix, five cans of tuna or chicken (or your preferred choice of protein), a container of feta, a bag of sunflower seeds, a pint of cherry tomatoes, and/or whatever other items you like to eat in a salad.

3. Put all five containers on the counter. Then, put one container on a kitchen scale. Put a portion of the salad mix into the container and write down how much it weighs.

(The reason you want to weigh each ingredient is because you need to be able to calculate exactly how many calories are in the salad. By checking the serving size weight on the bag of salad or container of feta, and how many calories are in a serving, you can figure out how many calories you are putting into your salad. Using an app like MyFitnessPal is very helpful, as you can create a recipe within the app that will calculate the calories for you.)

4. Split the rest of the salad mix evenly into the other containers.

5. Now put a tablespoon of sunflower seeds in each container, and write down 'A tablespoon of sunflowers'.

6. Split the pint of cherry tomatoes into five piles, and put one pile into each container. Write down how many cherry tomatoes went into each container.

7. Figure out how much feta you want in each salad; check the calories on the container and decide how many calories of feta you want. Weigh out the amount you want, so that you are certain of the calories. Again, check the weight of a serving of feta and how many calories it contains, so you can calculate how much you are putting in. Put that amount in each container, and write down how much feta went in.

8. Write down how many calories are in a can of tuna/chicken/protein and add that to your salad calorie list.

(You should now have a list that looks something like this... Salad: 150 grams, sunflower seeds: one tablespoon, cherry tomatoes: five pieces, feta: fifty grams. All you need to do now is input these amounts into a calorie counter like MyFitnessPal, or you can do the math yourself by looking up the calories for each ingredient.)

9. Each morning, grab a can of tuna/chicken/protein, a container of salad, and take them to work.

10. At lunchtime, add the protein to the salad and enjoy.

How long do you think that would take you on a Sunday afternoon? I would bet no longer than thirty minutes. You didn't even need to cut a single vegetable; a six-year-old could have prepared that salad. If you have kids, why not get them to help you and turn it into an activity with them?

Of course, most people don't want to live off salads alone (that would get pretty boring!). So, the second example shows you how to prepare a hot meal.

PREPARING A HOT MEAL

1. Buy five containers from a homewares store, as well as a food steamer.

2. Go to the grocery store and buy a tray of chicken thighs, a bag of pre-cut broccoli, and three instant rice packs (whatever flavour you like). Buy some sort of spice you like, whether it's chilli, paprika, shish kebab, jerk, or something else.

3. At home, preheat your oven to 350 °F, open the chicken pack, and cover the chicken in the spice of your choice. Put the chicken on a tray and cook for twenty minutes or however long is necessary.

4. While the chicken cooks, set up the steamer, and fill it with water. Put as much broccoli as you need for five meals into the steamer and cook it for about ten minutes.

5. Put the first rice pack into the microwave for two minutes, and repeat with the other rice packs.

6. Set up five containers. Put three cooked chicken thighs in each container, split the steamed broccoli into five portions and put them into the containers, and do the same with the rice.

7. Write down the calories in all three items (the chicken, rice and broccoli) so that you know how many calories are in each meal. To figure out how many calories are in each, check the nutritional facts label on the rice and chicken, and weigh the broccoli to calculate the calories. You can use Google or MyFitnessPal to find out how many calories are in a gram of broccoli and then multiply that by how many grams you have.

8. Put the containers in the fridge once cooled.

9. Take each container to work, microwave for two minutes and eat. Or enjoy at dinnertime.

This meal is super healthy, super cheap, and requires no fuss. You could do this in thirty minutes, no problem.

These are just two simple examples I wanted to give you to get your brain ticking over. When you see it broken down like that, you realize it's not hard at all. Now, I know no one really wants to spend their Sunday afternoon meal prepping, but it's a great way to build discipline. You're creating this great habit at the start of your week, which is the perfect way to get you into the mindset of staying on track for the whole week. Remember, building discipline requires some discomfort, so suck it up, prep some meals, and enjoy the satisfaction of knowing that whatever happens at work this week, at least you have a healthy lunch or dinner you can turn to when your life gets hectic.

FOUR POPULAR DIETS

There are so many diets out there that it's hard to know if one is better than the other. Ketogenic, intermittent fasting, paleo, and low-fat or low-carb are just some of the buzz diets that people are attempting to follow right now. Here's a quick breakdown of what each one does.

The Ketogenic Diet

The ketogenic, or keto, diet is a low-carb, high-fat diet. It lowers blood sugar and insulin levels, and shifts the body's metabolism away from carbs and toward fat and ketones. When this happens, your body becomes incredibly efficient at burning fat for energy. It also turns fat into ketones in the liver, which can supply energy for the brain. Note: it is super restrictive. If you happen to eat some sort of food that has the smallest amount of sugar in it, you will come out of ketosis (the metabolic state caused by the keto diet) and you won't be burning fat efficiently.

Intermittent Fasting

Intermittent fasting is the process of cycling in and out of periods of eating and not eating. Although people do experience weight loss with intermittent fasting, it is less of a diet plan and more of a lifestyle choice, focusing on *when* you eat, not *what* you eat. There are a few different ways that people do intermittent fasting. Typically, most people will fast for twelve to sixteen hours a day, while others eat normally for five days and reduce their calories down to 600 or so on the other two days.

The Paleo Diet

The paleo diet is based on foods that are thought to have existed in the Paleolithic era, some 10,000-plus years ago. This includes fish, lean meats, vegetables, fruits, nuts and seeds. In other words, food that would have been collected through hunting and gathering. Foods that aren't eaten are things like grains, legumes, dairy products, sugar, or any processed foods.

Low-Fat and Low-Carb Diets

Low-fat or low-carb diets are exactly what they sound like – diets that consist of eating foods that have minimal fat or carbs. These diets are often quite similar to some of the other diets. For example, a low-carb diet is quite similar to the paleo diet. To eat low-carb, you would have to avoid food like rice, bread, sugar and grains, which is basically the same as the paleo diet.

PICKING A DIET THAT WORKS FOR YOU

Now that we have covered the most common diets out there, you're probably wondering which one will give you the quickest – and best – results. You may be thinking, 'Just tell me which one to follow and I'll do it.' If only it was that easy! If there was one diet that actually did what you wanted, and worked without fail, then everyone would be following it. What if I told you that all the diets mentioned in the previous section are essentially doing the exact same thing? If anyone loses weight on any of these diets, it's because they were in a calorie deficit (more calories out than in). It wasn't because of the diet specifically; it was because of the deficit.

However, you have to pay attention to exactly *what* you're eating so that you're less likely to overeat. For example, if you are following a low-carb diet, you need to pay attention to every bit of food you're eating to determine whether it is a carb or not. That's going to force you to eat more vegetables than you normally would, as vegetables are lower in carbs than, say, rice or pasta. Also, you may discover that all the snacks you've been buying have sugar and carbs in them, so you'll stop eating them, which means by osmosis you'll stop eating as much during the day, which in turn will cause you to lose weight.

The same goes for intermittent fasting. If you normally eat breakfast and then a snack at 10 a.m., and then lunch at 12:00 p.m., by 1:00 p.m. you've potentially already eaten 1,500 calories or more. By fasting until 1:00 p.m., you're missing out on eating all that food. If you then break your fast and have a big lunch, it's highly unlikely that you're going to eat those extra 1,500 calories in the afternoon. So, again, by not overeating, you might start to lose some weight.

The takeaway message here is that there really isn't any specific diet that is better than the other. Obviously, any diet that consists of natural, unprocessed foods, ideally without hormones and pesticides, is going to be the best for you. We all know that. By 'unprocessed foods', I mean things like meats, fish, grains, vegetables, fruits, nuts and seeds. Here's an easy way to determine if something is a natural, unprocessed food: if you pick up the package and read the list of ingredients, and there are things you can't pronounce or don't know what they are, that means that particular food item is processed and has chemicals and other agents in it.

Think of a diet as a tool you can use, not as a black-and-white rule you have to follow. Most people let their diet control them, but that doesn't work. Remember, *you* have to be in control, so let your diet work for you. I know some people who religiously follow a vegan diet who are in terrible shape and health. I also know some who are in amazing shape and they love it.

I know some people who religiously follow the keto diet, who never get to enjoy a sugary treat, never get to eat outside of the keto box, and they hate it. I know people who love keto because of that very reason; it's so restrictive that it forces them to not eat junk food or sugar. The point is, what works for me might not work for you. And ultimately, if I'm in charge of my life choices, then whatever diet I follow should give me the results I want. (As long as I'm not eating more calories than I'm burning, right?)

Before we wrap up this chapter on nutrition, I'll share with you what my current eating habits are, so that you can see how I treat 'dieting' as a tool versus something set in stone. Now remember, this is my personal opinion and routine of what I think works best for my specific goals, so this kind of protocol might not be suitable for you and your goals. However, I think it's important for you to understand how I think about and control my eating habits. I have a few rules that I follow, which create boundaries and structure for me, which suits my personality and my long-term life goals.

JAY'S NUTRITION ROUTINE

1. Never deny myself food I want, but also never deny the impact that food will have on my calorie count, energy and health. This means that if I decide that I want to eat a donut, I eat a donut, but I don't pretend that the donut isn't covered in sugar, that it doesn't contain 500 calories, or that it's at all good for me. Every time I think about eating something unhealthy, this simple reminder can be enough to steer me away from the craving.

2. Always keep a mental note of how many calories I've eaten for the day, Sunday to Friday. On Saturdays, I usually just eat as much as I feel like. (This is the eighty per cent rule we covered earlier in the book.)

3. On public holidays, long weekends or holidays, I eat whatever I want; it's my time to enjoy anything I want. (I know I have to apply discipline as soon as the holiday is over in order to get straight back to my normal eating patterns.)

4. If I decided to indulge myself during the week to fulfill a craving, the next food choice always needs to be a better option. For example, if I have a burger and fries for lunch, that means dinner has to be a healthy, nutritious meal. I don't want to eat

unhealthy meals back to back, because I don't want to overeat that day and I don't want my body to be filled with garbage.

In terms of my actual diet, I like to switch from diet to diet and take what I like from each of them. I typically will do intermittent fasting every day until at least 10:00 a.m. and sometimes until 1:00 p.m., depending on what my day is like. I used to eat my first meal at 5:00 a.m. (I'm an early riser!). By the time 10:00 a.m. came around, I was often eating a full meal again, and by 1:00 p.m. I had eaten three full meals. In short, I was eating too much food.

When I break my fast, my first meal is usually a keto meal, meaning high-fat and no sugar or carbs. Since I've been fasting for fourteen to sixteen hours, my body has burnt up all the food from the day before and is now in fat-burning mode. I like to fuel my body with more fats and keep it in ketosis, so that it will continue to burn fat for the next few hours until my next meal.

Typically, I work out in the afternoon, around 3:00 p.m. So, depending on my workout, I have some protein and a small amount of carbs to fuel my body. When it comes to my last meal of the day, I like to eat a really big meal, with lots of protein, lots of vegetables and carbs. I have the biggest portion of food for the day as my dinner. Why? Because I know I like to snack after dinner and it's never anything healthy. So, if I eat a big meal for dinner, I'm going to be full and unlikely to want to snack after.

Notice how I'm eating very specifically for my schedule and to reflect my personal habits? This doesn't mean this is completely set in stone. For example, if a friend asks me to meet them for brunch on the weekend, it doesn't mean I don't eat because I'm fasting; I adapt and change things up.

On days like that, I'll go eat a big brunch, and enjoy myself with my friend, but then I might not eat again until the evening. And if my brunch was very high in carbs, I might make my evening meal lighter, with fewer carbs and more vegetables. I also might make my evening meal smaller. But since it's the weekend, I'll probably want to eat some treats after dinner. See how I'm reacting to my daily situation and adjusting accordingly? You can do the same.

CHAPTER SUMMARY

Following a strict diet that is set in stone is almost impossible. And as soon as you (inevitably) break the diet, you end up just giving up completely and going back to square one, where you're not paying attention to any of your eating habits. Paying attention to, and understanding the impact of, the food you eat is how you win your Personal Revolution. That's why it's so important to educate yourself about nutrition, but also create a nutritional routine that is realistic and easy to maintain.

7

EXERCISE

Now that you know that nutrition is the number one tool to change your body composition, particularly if you are trying to lose some body fat, it's time to complete the final step in the Personal Revolution process: 'Exercise'.

I want you to gain a new appreciation for exercise and working out. Instead of doing workouts you might hate because you think they are going to help you lose weight, now you will pick workouts that you do purely for enjoyment, or for other goals such as building muscle, getting stronger, gaining more or better movement, improving your skill level in a particular sport, or improving your coordination.

In this chapter, I'm going to explain the major kinds of workouts you could choose to do and why you would choose them. I'll also explain how you can work out on your own to save time and to ensure you don't miss an opportunity to do something physical. We'll also cover how to pick a gym and a trainer, and how to create a long-term fitness plan to keep you interested and dedicated.

FIVE TYPES OF FITNESS TRAINING

There are different kinds of workouts you can do, and each one gives you different results.

Understanding each is important because you can then pick the kind of workout you want to be doing, according to your goals or interests.

Strength, cardiovascular, flexibility, balance and agility are the five major types of fitness training you can do. I think it is important to make sure that you are incorporating a little bit of each type into your overall routine, so that long term you are physically well rounded. However, in terms of creating your short-term fitness goals and giving yourself something to work toward, you need to pick something that falls under one of those categories, which you're able to measure your improvement off. So, with that in mind, here's an overview of each type of fitness training.

Strength

Strength training is exactly what it sounds like – building strength in your body. Strength can mean something different for everyone. Maybe it means being able to carry your kids on your back while you go for a walk. It can mean being able to do a two-plate squat and deadlift. It can mean you're focusing on building muscle so that you're more muscular and athletic in appearance.

Strength training is what most people are doing in the gym when you think of a typical gym workout. When you're in the gym lifting weights, this is strength training. Strength training is known to be great for building muscle, improving posture, bone density and joint stability, and reducing everyday injuries. The most common kind of strength exercises are things like squats, deadlifts, push-ups, bicep curls, shoulder presses, chest presses and lunges, to name a few.

Cardiovascular

Cardiovascular training, by definition, is 'physical conditioning that exercises the heart, lungs and associated blood vessels'. You can tell just by the definition how important cardiovascular training (or cardio, as it's commonly called) is for you. There is no right way to do cardio. You're going to read and hear all sorts of conflicting information, such as you need to do it for at least twenty-five minutes, or you need to keep your heart rate up the whole time, or you need to do it slow, or fast, or it has to be done three times a week. *All* this information is correct, depending on why you're doing cardio in the first place.

Like most things in life, look back at the definition of what it is, and, if what you're doing matches it, then you're doing it. So as long as you are doing some sort of physical activity that 'exercises the heart', which means your heart rate is higher than normal, and 'exercises the lungs and associated blood vessels', which means you are breathing heavier than you normally would, then that's cardio and you're doing it!

Anything beyond that should be determined by what your goals are. If you are trying to lose a lot of weight, then you might want to do a lot of cardio, focusing on keeping your heart rate within the fat-burning zone. If you want to get better at playing a particular sport, you might want to focus on doing short bursts of fast cardio to simulate what happens in the game. If you want to be able to run your first five-kilometre race, then doing running as your cardio makes sense.

The point is, until you know what your goals are, and what you are trying to achieve, it doesn't matter what cardio you decide to do. Some of the most common cardio exercises are things like running, biking, walking, swimming, dancing, aerobics and rowing.

Flexibility

Flexibility training refers to developing a wide range of motion in a joint or series of joints, which is attained by using equipment or through brief amounts of physical effort. It not only refers to the movement of joints – it also refers to the muscle mobility around the joints. Range of motion is the distance and direction your joints can move, while mobility is the ability to move without restriction.

The older you get, the more and more valuable flexibility training is going to become to you. Personally, being able to walk upstairs, or comfortably bend my knees and hips to get in and out of a chair, is super important to me. However, this doesn't mean you should just wait until you're older to start flexibility training. On the contrary, you need to start now. Once your joints and muscles are locked up, it's going to be a lot harder to get them moving again. In this way, think of flexibility training like constantly keeping your joints oiled.

Doing some sort of flexibility training, regardless of how old you are, is important. You don't need to become a yoga guru. Perhaps just a well-thought-out stretch routine a couple of times a week is enough for you. Some common workouts that are considered flexibility training are things like yoga, Pilates, tai chi, Animal Flow (a structured series of animal-style movements that can be linked together to form flows, similar to yoga) and ELDOA (which stands for – wait for it – Elongation Longitudinaux Avec Decoaption Osteo Articulaire). ELDOA is a system of exercises designed to ease pain, boost circulation, and improve posture, balance, and spine health.

Balance and Agility

I've combined balance and agility training together because they are often done at the same time. Balance is something that you probably don't care too much about now, but, again, it's something to be more concerned about as you get older. This includes things like getting in and out of a shower, steadying yourself if someone accidentally bumps into you at the mall, and walking on an uneven surface. However, it isn't just important to have good balance when you're old. If you want to play any kind of sport or want to improve your athletic ability, then balance is super important. This is where it goes hand in hand with agility training.

Agility is the ability to move quickly and easily – being able to stop, start and change directions quickly when needed. Pretty much any sport you can think of requires some level of agility, and a sense of balance. Being able to move freely in different directions is super important, even if you have no intention of ever playing a sport. Think of running upstairs around people, moving quickly through a subway station, jumping out of the way to avoid a car splashing water on you, and so on. These are all examples of using your agility in everyday life.

The most common way to train for improved balance and agility is to participate in any sort of fitness class you like. Be it boxing, boot camps, HIIT (high-intensity interval training), body pump, or cardio kickboxing, these will all have an element of balance and agility in them. If you don't want to do a class and want to train on your own, then things like ladder drills, cone drills, Bosu ball exercises, and single leg exercises (like step-ups, walking lunges, and pistol squats) are very common exercises you could be doing.

HOW TO WORK OUT ON YOUR OWN

Although this is just a small section of the book, I consider this to be probably the most important information I want to give you if you don't know how to work out on your own. I'll be perfectly blunt and say that unless you learn how to do this, any Personal Revolution you attempt to win will not be successful.

I couldn't give you a more perfect example of why this is true than the COVID-19 pandemic, which forced much of the world into lockdown to slow down the spread of the virus. For a time, gyms everywhere closed their doors. Anyone who relied solely on a trainer or fitness studio for their workouts was suddenly thrown completely off course. Some people stopped working out altogether, as their whole routine was thrown off.

For some people, it will take months or even years to get back on the wagon, long after the gyms and fitness studios reopen in full. As for my clients, I'm not worried about them at all. I've taught them how to work out on their own, so they don't rely on me 100 per cent of the time. I've sent them all workouts they can do at home, without any equipment, and I know they are going to do them.

I want you to take working out on your own seriously. It's a skill you must learn as part of looking after yourself. That's not to say that you shouldn't hire a trainer or join a fitness program. In fact, you should definitely be doing something like that. Just make sure all your eggs aren't in one basket. Only you and you alone can be responsible for your health and wellbeing. So, with that in mind, here are some tips to help you get started.

Take Ownership of Your Fitness

Working out on your own is all about the mindset you have going into it. It doesn't matter what app you're using or which workout you are doing. It's about you taking ownership of your own fitness. One of the biggest mistakes people make when they try to start working out on their own is trying to find the best app, the best program, and so on.

I can't tell you the number of times I've heard, 'I want to start working out but I don't know what to search for or what the best website is to learn.' Guess what? It doesn't matter. Learning is learning. It would be like saying, 'I've always wanted to learn Spanish, but I didn't know which "learn to speak Spanish book" to buy, so I never started.' That's kind of foolish, right?

Make Use of YouTube, Apps and Online Programs

The great thing about today's online society is that there are so many resources you can tap into for free or for little cost. One place to start feeling comfortable doing something on your own is YouTube. Set up some space in your living room and search for pretty much any kind of workout you can imagine, and you will find it on YouTube. Yoga, boot camp, boxercise, stretching, strength training – it's all there.

If you would like something more structured, with more of a progression element to it, then look to your smartphone for a fitness app. Again, any kind of workout you can imagine, you can find on there. This includes 'learn to run' apps, 'how to get six-pack abs' apps, weight loss apps, yoga apps, and more. Again, it's all there, often free or for a small price.

And lastly, you can simply search the internet for any kind of workout you want to learn, and there are millions of websites with information on how to do it. Most of the information you can find for free, or for a small cost you can sign up to a platform or membership site, which will provide you with workouts and programs to follow.

Remember the point of working out on your own is to *figure out* working out on your own, so I want you to apply some caution when signing up to any sort of program. Make sure you aren't just relying on it to give you the information and workouts. What happens if that program suddenly disappears? Have you actually learned how to work out on your own or were you just following along?

Pick Body Weight Exercises

The first place you should start when trying to create a workout on your own is to pick body weight exercises. This means you don't need any equipment; you're just using your own body weight. These are great because most body weight exercises use multiple muscle groups at once, so they are very effective in getting your whole body moving.

If you want to break it down a little further, then break down the exercises into primary movements so that you can make sure you are covering all the movements that we use in everyday life. Squatting, lunging, pushing, pulling and rotating are the most common movements we make. If you look at that list of movements, you can pretty much create a workout just from looking at the names. Squats, lunges, push-ups, pull-ups, rotating plank – there's a workout.

Determine the Number of Reps and Sets

Once you have your workout, all you need to do is figure out how many reps and how many sets you are going to do. Again, there is no right answer to this question – it depends on what you are trying to achieve. However, if you are just starting out, then a good place to start is doing ten to fifteen reps per exercise and three to four sets of each. Ideally, you want to pair up the exercises into groups of two or three, so that you move back and forth from one to the other. You don't have to, but it's an efficient way to make sure that you are moving consistently throughout your workout, and you can rest one group of muscles while you work the others.

YOUR HYPOTHETICAL WORKOUT

To put it all together, it might look something like this:

1. Squats: ten reps (working legs).

2. Push-ups: ten reps (working chest and triceps).

3. Repeat the previous steps three times.

1. Lunges: fourteen reps (working legs).

2. Pull-ups: ten reps (working back and biceps).

3. Rotating plank: twelve reps (working core and abs).

4. Repeat the previous steps three times.

As you get more confident, look for more body weight exercises you can do on your own and start adding those to your routine. Don't overthink it – it's better for you to do something than nothing.

HOW TO PICK A GYM, STUDIO OR TRAINER

This is quite a common question for a lot of people, so I think it's worth addressing in case it's something that you wonder about as well. There are a few key elements you need to consider when picking a gym or trainer. (For simplicity, I'm going to refer to both gyms and studios as 'gyms'. However, by 'studio', I mean anywhere that holds fitness classes, be it yoga, boxing, boot camp, or spinning, to name a few.)

Don't overlook any of them because you don't want to be part of the eighty per cent of people who have a gym membership and don't use it consistently. Or who quit in the first six months. According to the 2019 IHRSA Health Club Consumer Report, only eighteen per cent of gym members use the gym consistently. What's more, the majority of health clubs and gyms lose fifty per cent of their new members within the first six months.

With that in mind, here are some tips to help you pick the right gym, studio or trainer.

Be Mindful of the Distance From Your House or Workplace

Don't pick a gym that is too far from your house or your workplace. The reality is that even if you pick the best gym in the city, if you have to spend forty minutes commuting to get there, you aren't going to go. Chances are, if you're working a corporate job like most of my clients are, you really only have two, possibly three, options in terms of times you can work out:

- Before work (between 5:30 a.m. and 8:00 a.m.),
- After work (5:00 p.m. to 8:00 p.m.), and
- Possibly in your lunch break. (Ninety per cent of my clients don't even take a lunch break, but, in theory, if the gym were close enough, you could duck out for a quick thirty-minute workout.)

So, pick a gym that you can get to easily on your way to or from work. It should take you no longer than fifteen minutes to get there. This eliminates the excuse of not having enough time to get to the gym.

Check What Facilities the Gym Has

Make sure the gym you are looking at joining has all the facilities you actually want and need. If you plan on working out before work and the gym doesn't have showers, then do you have enough time to go home and shower before you go to work? A lot of smaller gyms don't have showers so, although they can be great places to work out, I personally don't think it's smart to eliminate one of the few opportunities in the day you have to work out. Sometimes things change at work. If suddenly you have to stay back every day to finish a project, and you can't work out in the mornings, guess what happens to your workout routine? It doesn't happen.

Also check that you aren't going to be paying for facilities that you aren't going to use. For example, I know of a high-end gym that includes a café, a salad bar, and even an alcohol service – things I would never use when I go to the gym. I'm not saying these aren't useful services, but personally I don't want to pay for a premium venue if I'm not going to use at least sixty per cent of the services.

Finally, it's all the little details that are going to keep you interested and motivated to go, so be sure to consider those. Check that the showers have free soap, shampoo, and so on. Note how clean the gym is. Does it offer a towel service, and is this included with your membership? Are there lockers where you can store your stuff and do you need to bring your own lock? Is there cold drinking water available? What are the opening and closing hours? If it's a studio, what is the schedule like? Does it line up with your work schedule, so you can go regularly?

See how all these little things could really impact your workout routine if they don't all line up with what you actually want? I personally don't want to have to carry a towel, a bottle of water and a lock with me all the time when I go to the gym, because I often decide to go spur of the moment when I have some time.

Search for Reviews and Recommendations
As with anything, ask around. If you're looking for a gym or trainer

that's accessible to your workplace, then check with your work colleagues and they will be able to give you some recommendations. If you're lucky, you might have just found yourself a workout partner while asking around. Or at least someone you can walk to the gym with because, as we covered earlier, having someone else to go with increases the likelihood of being consistent tenfold.

When asking around for recommendations, make sure you ask some specific questions to help find the kind of gym or trainer you are looking for. Particularly when picking a trainer, ask questions like:

- Why specifically do you recommend them?
- What results have you achieved with them?
- What have you learned from them?

Dig a little bit deeper – make sure they aren't just saying things like, 'Oh, my trainer is great. We have a fun time.' Or, in contrast to that, 'The workouts are really hard.' You need to get past the subjective answers and into the specifics of what makes them a good trainer. I would want to know things like:

- Do they ask you about your goals and then create a plan that aligns with them?
- Do they track and measure your results?
- Do they help you create routines and habits you can maintain on your own?

See how you could start to tell whether the trainer was worth contacting or not by asking those kinds of questions?

Finally, go online and look at reviews to see what everyone else is saying about a gym or trainer. Google any of my fitness businesses and I hope you see five-star reviews across the board. Don't just look at the stars though. Read the reviews, spend some time going back through them all, and check to see whether they look legitimate or not. Unfortunately, often when a gym or trainer gets a few bad reviews, they ask their friends to go add a bunch of positive reviews and it hides the bad ones. Check reviews across multiple sites, such as Google, Facebook, Yelp, and so on, to make sure the messaging is consistent.

Verify Credentials and Experience

Don't overlook this step in finding a gym or trainer, but more so a trainer. I'm always surprised when someone reaches out to work with me, but they never ask any questions like:

- Do you have insurance? (This is important for two reasons. Firstly, if you get seriously injured, your trainer's insurance might cover your medical bills. Secondly, in order for a trainer to get insurance, they need to keep their personal training certifications up to date. This means they have been continually educating themselves, as this is a requirement to renew PT certifications.)
- What new courses or workshops have you done recently?
- Have you continued your health and fitness education since becoming a personal trainer?
- What are some client results that you are most proud of?

These questions will put a trainer on the spot and force them off their normal sales pitch, so you can get a bit of insight into what they are really like. For example, asking a trainer what new courses they have done recently isn't so much about the courses themselves. It's more about finding out whether this person continues to educate themselves as a health and fitness professional. Best practices and exercise science are always changing. Personally, I want to work with someone who is up to date with the industry.

Don't be afraid to ask some intimate and challenging questions as well. You could ask questions like:

- What sort of people don't you like working with, and why?
- What is your training style? Are you extremely strict, or are you relaxed?
- When was the last time you pushed yourself out of your comfort zone?
- Have you recently achieved some sort of physical goal?
- Have you ever been overweight or lost a lot of weight?

Remember, you're about to put a lot of trust in this person. You're expecting them to train you properly in an environment where you could get injured, and to make recommendations about your health and body, which should be best suited to you and your goals. You want to know what sort of trainer they are, and whether they're suited to you. Will they inspire you to achieve your goals? Do you share any common interests or views? You should put a lot of thought into this decision.

Here's a case study featuring one of my clients, Heba, who explains why he chose me as his trainer.

HEBA'S STORY

'I met Jay at a time when I was seeking a very specific kind of training experience. As a former semi-professional athlete, my relationship with personal training and athletic coaching is complicated. Although I have been working through this with a dedicated yoga practice, I still felt something was lacking, particularly when it came to preventing injury. I needed a particular type of targeted physical and mental conditioning, but I didn't even know where to start looking for it.

'Fortunately, I crossed paths with Jay in our building's gym and my decision to work with him was a highly intuitive experience. As I observed him train a neighbour, there was something about his demeanour, vitality, and deliberate creativity that compelled me to reach out. Within minutes of communication, I knew he was the trainer I was looking for and I hired him on the spot.

'From that point onwards began a deeply gratifying experience, guided by Jay's gentle questions and careful reflections. Although we spent time discussing my history, Jay was determined to keep the focus on how I wanted my body to feel today and in the future. I saw results in the studio almost immediately. More importantly, Jay understood and respected my desire to stay injury free and observed me very closely, always listening for cues and absorbing what I wanted for myself in order to reflect it back to me.

'With his deep understanding of the body and mind, he helped me self-realize in a way that had been eluding me for years.

I learned things about myself which continue to aid me as I navigate the next stages of my life. This journey was about more than physical conditioning. It was about relearning a relationship with my physical and mental self to further deepen my yoga practice and way of life. I found the perfect collaborator in Jay and his Personal Revolution program.'

CREATING SUSTAINABLE, LONG-TERM FITNESS PLANS

Now that you know the different kinds of workouts you can do, how to work out, and how to pick a gym or a trainer, all you need to do is create a fitness plan you can stick with long term. Here are some ways to help you do that.

Align Your Fitness Plan With Your Goals

If you think back to the start of the book, in Step 1: Clarity, I suggested breaking down your goals into daily, weekly, monthly, quarterly, and half yearly goals. So, make sure that, first and foremost, your fitness plan aligns with the goals you have. It would be a bit stupid to have a weekly goal of working out four times, but a fitness plan that had a three-day weight training routine. Every week you would be trying to figure out what your fourth workout was going to be. So, make sure that the fitness plan you have in place is helping you achieve your goals in the most efficient way possible.

If your quarterly goal is to run a ten-kilometre race and your fitness plan doesn't include running, then you have a problem. I know you're thinking, 'Yeah, of course. Why wouldn't I be running if my goal was to do a ten-kilometre race?' But believe me, this mismatch of goal to fitness plan happens all the time, so much so that I have to mention it.

As humans, we have a strange way of changing our goals and desires, but forgetting to change our behaviour to match. Think back over your life to a time when you had an activity as part of your routine, only to suddenly realize, 'Wow, I don't even like doing this anymore. Why am I doing this?'

That happened to me. I was sitting in a bar on a Friday night when I suddenly realized, 'I don't even like doing this – I'm bored.' The funny thing is, I probably figured that out six months too late. I had changed, but my behaviour hadn't. Make sure your goals and your fitness plan are in a constant feedback loop with each other, so that you stay motivated and the workouts you do are always working toward a bigger picture. You're going to feel like you have a purpose, a mission, every time you work out. As soon as you lose your purpose, your reason to work out, your Personal Revolution is doomed.

GREG'S STORY

A common example of keeping goals and fitness plans in alignment, even when one of them changes, is when a client comes to me wanting to lose weight. Take my long-term client Greg, a pharmacist whose original goal was to lose twenty to thirty pounds of body fat. I set up a specific workout plan for him that included guidelines for the number of calories per day he should eat, the kind of workouts he should be doing, and how many times a week he should be working out.

In short, his fitness plan was aligned to his goal of losing weight. Greg had 'Clarity' on what his goal was, we 'Measured' his results every six weeks, he had 'Discipline' to work out regularly, his 'Nutrition' was to eat fewer calories than he burnt during the week, and his 'Exercise' was to run twice a week and do circuit training three times a week.

The plan worked and over time he lost the weight he wanted. However, it came to a point where I had to sit down with him and get him to question whether his goals were actually still the same, or whether they had changed. He was so focused on losing weight that he wasn't really recognizing that he'd achieved this goal and that it was time to change gears. His real goal now was to gain muscle and shape his body.

In other words, he had changed but hadn't realized it yet. Eventually, his whole fitness plan changed to reflect – and help him achieve – his new goals. It was quite an 'aha!' moment for him to suddenly see the shift he had made in his mindset and goals without even realizing.

Break It Down Into Six-Week Blocks

The best way to create a sustainable plan is to run your fitness routines in six-week blocks and then reassess. Create a plan, commit to it for six weeks, and then take a minute to ask yourself questions like:

- Is this working?
- Am I enjoying this?
- Are my goals still the same?
- Have I adapted to this fitness plan and do I need to make it harder?

- Do I want to keep doing the same routine or do I want to change it up?

These questions are part of the feedback loop between your fitness plan and your overall goals. I don't always change my clients' fitness plans every six weeks, but I always ask these questions. Often the plan is working really well, they are enjoying it, they are getting results and they are motivated to continue, so we run the same plan for another six weeks. Then we reassess again. The point is to stop and take note of how you feel and to check in on yourself.

If your goal is to simply start finding time in your busy schedule to work out, then your fitness plan could be to commit to working out twice a week for the next six weeks. That's a good plan. Commit to that and, in six weeks, look back at how it's been. Maybe now you're in a great routine and you want to try to work out three times a week. Commit to three times a week for the next six weeks, and maybe get a trainer to help you create an interesting routine to keep you motivated.

Don't Overthink It

Finally, creating a long-term plan shouldn't be complicated, so don't overthink it. Like pretty much everything else in this book, all I want you to do is pay attention to what you are doing and exercise with intention. If you just commit to exercising and that's good enough for you, then that's your intention and I'm happy with that.

Over the years, I've worked with dozens of executives who have come to me and said, 'Jay, the fact that I'm here working out is enough of a challenge for me, so please don't ask me to follow any routines on my own or any diet, or do extra homework, as I'm not going to be able do it.' I respect that, and appreciate they are at least taking control of their health by doing *something*. Sometimes it's taken them a whole lifetime to get themselves into a gym, so I applaud them for that.

As long as you have a plan – any plan – you are moving in the right direction. Your job and your career are complicated enough, so make your fitness plan as simple and as easy to follow as possible.

CHAPTER SUMMARY

Exercise doesn't have to be all about losing weight or getting into 'shape'. There are many ways you can exercise and each of them will give you different results. Some of the most common ways are strength, cardio, flexibility, balance and agility. Understanding that each kind of exercise achieves a different result is crucial for your short- and long-term fitness goals. Pick workouts that complement your goals so that you achieve the results you actually want.

One of the most important aspects of exercise is being able to do it on your own. You won't be able to win your Personal Revolution if you can't nail this part of it. By all means, use a trainer or join a fitness program to help you, but ultimately you still have to do the work. They can't work out for you. If you don't know where to begin, then body weight exercises are a good starting point.

When it comes time to progress a bit further, and you want to find a trainer or a gym, remember to choose carefully. Above all, don't overthink exercise. Something is always better than nothing. As long as you have a plan to follow, the rest will fall into place.

CONCLUSION

YOUR LIFE, YOUR POTENTIAL, YOUR REVOLUTION

I'm guessing by now you're ready to drop this book, so you can get started on mapping out your strategic plan to fight and win your Personal Revolution. I'm hoping you don't feel overwhelmed by the idea of all this change, but are excited to finally achieve a balance between having a career and having the body, health and fitness you've always wanted.

There is no reason why you should be sacrificing that whole part of your life to get ahead at work. Now that you know that everything in your life is based around your health and fitness, that should be even more motivation for you to get a handle on it. And you can be sure you'll reap the rewards as a result. You think you're successful now? Just wait until you're fit, sharp, healthy, feeling good, and looking good. Your productivity and energy will go through the roof.

TONYA'S STORY

Tonya came to me as a burnt out, overweight, broken and exhausted CEO of a prominent social innovation company here in Toronto. She told me straight from the start she hated sweating, hated working out in groups, and was struggling to get her personal health and life in order due to massive work and social commitments. Boy, I had my work cut out for me.

I decided that the best approach in Tonya's case was to work with her one-on-one using the framework from my Personal Revolution Fast-Track Program, which I designed specifically for clients who require more hands-on attention from me. Guess what the very first thing we did was? If you guessed the Clarity exercise from chapter two, then you would be correct.

We spent two hours working through her beliefs, her vision, her purpose, and her strategy. We underlined all the things she wanted and all the things she wouldn't get if she didn't act, all the things she could change, and all the things she *wanted* to change. By the end, we had uncovered enough pain points and enough inspiration to get her motivated and on board with achieving her Personal Revolution, doing it right and, this time, making it permanent.

What came next? Measurements, of course. I recorded all the measurements that I mentioned in chapter four: BFP, weight, and body measurements. I made sure we had a record of all that, so that we could track her progress when we came back to re-measure.

Tonya already had quite a good morning routine in place, but I was able to improve her routine by giving her access to my daily coaching and tracking app, which is designed to improve your discipline. It does this by reminding you to do your workouts, to do your daily check-in with yourself, and to stay focused on your short-term goals as you ramp up your health and fitness routines. By keeping track each day of how she slept, how much energy she had, how much exercise she was doing, and how her stress levels were, she was able to become more disciplined. This helped her stick to the things that were improving her life, and remove things that were having negative impacts.

A perfect example of this was recording which nights she drank alcohol and which nights she didn't sleep well. By doing this, she was able to make the connection that every time she had more than a glass of wine, she didn't sleep well. She implemented one of the Personal Revolution rules of 'One night a week', and, within a week, she was sleeping better than she had in years. Imagine that. If you just reduced your alcohol consumption down to twenty per cent, you could be having the best night's sleep you've had in years. It's food for thought, isn't it?

Speaking of food, next I looked at Tonya's nutrition. She had been on and off all sorts of diets, most recently a keto diet. She'd had great success on it in the past, but it wasn't working for her anymore. She was extremely frustrated at the extra weight she was carrying and at her failure to lose any of it, even while she was trying so hard to be 'good' by sticking to her diet. I analyzed her food intake and how many calories a day she was burning, and I was able to determine that she was undereating significantly. Her body was in extreme starvation mode and out of whack from drinking too much booze, being on and off keto, and managing her nutrition poorly for months.

So instead of going on a diet, she actually needed to focus on eating more food, and a more balanced variety of foods, to get her body used to burning more energy and fire up her metabolism again. Notice how I measured first, then interpreted that data based on what was happening in her life to make a plan that was appropriate for her? I didn't just put her on a generic weight loss diet because that was *her* immediate goal. The *real* immediate goal was to get her body functioning properly again with the right foods and right number of calories. One of the positive side effects of this was that it reduced a lot of the stress that was built up around trying to diet and eat in such a restricted way. Removing that stress around food enabled her body to adjust and make the changes it needed so that she felt great, and had way more energy. Although it took longer than she initially wanted, she was able to start losing weight while enjoying the food she liked without stress.

And finally, I needed to implement an exercise plan that she would be motivated to stick to and that she actually enjoyed. Remember she said she didn't like group classes or sweating? So, we had to get creative. Tonya was already doing a morning walk with her dog, so I decided to turn her morning walk into a workout as well. How? By giving her a selection of exercises that she could do along the route. For example, when she walked past a large rock, she could do step-ups on it. When she came across a park bench, she could do push-ups off it. When she found a set of stairs, she could run up them.

The idea was to build off the walking routine she already had, and make it fun and interesting so that it didn't feel like a traditional workout. I also created an at-home workout routine, which incorporated exercises that her chiropractor had given her: yoga moves, stretches, and some strength exercises using dumbbells. She absolutely loved this workout routine because she could feel that she was getting stronger, her body was moving a lot better due to the yoga and stretches, and she even began to enjoy getting a sweat on because she felt like the workout was perfect for her body and it made her feel great.

When it came time to redo Tonya's measurements, we found she had achieved massive improvements in reducing her body fat and her body size, and losing the weight she wanted. She was now comfortably working out three to four times a week, she had replaced most of her alcohol with teas and waters, and most of the little aches and pains she had been carrying for years had either completely gone or were significantly reduced. Most importantly, she felt fantastic, had reduced her stress tenfold, and was loving her new lease on life. She won her Personal Revolution!

I hope this story highlights the success of the five-step process, and how all you need to do is apply it to your own life, step by step. This isn't a rare example of what can be achieved by going through the steps. This is what I expect, and see time and time again, with every client I work with, either one-on-one or in my Personal Revolution Accelerator. Please, just follow the steps, the exercises and the rules, and experience the transformation that Tonya and many others have had before you. I want this for you too.

THE FIVE-STEP PROCESS IS READY AND WAITING

The strategies and processes described in this book aren't hard, and they aren't complicated. All you need to do is follow them step by step and in the order I've laid out for you. Here's a quick recap:

Step 1: Clarity
Don't make the common mistake of jumping into the Nutrition and Exercise steps before starting at Clarity, the first step in the Personal Revolution process. Remember, until you figure out your 'why', you're going to struggle with committing to this process. In fact, your chances of maintaining momentum past the initial honeymoon phase will be extremely slim, and very soon you'll be back where you started.

Go deep and find the 'why' that gives you a strong enough conviction that, from this moment forth, your health and fitness is the most important part of your life. Take a well-rounded, holistic approach to your Personal Revolution. Do it once and do it right. This is for life. Write down your rules of engagement so you don't forget them, but don't be too hard on yourself. Live at eighty per cent constantly – rather than 100 per cent only some of the time – and take advantage of the beauty of compound interest as your improvements keep stacking up on themselves.

Step 2: Measure
Don't forget to Measure – it's so important to be tracking your results and your progress. Nothing will keep you more motivated than seeing the scales change, or your body fat percentage go down. Likewise, for me personally, nothing gets me back on track quicker

than if I see my body fat has gone up, or the scale pops up a few pounds and I know I haven't been gaining muscle.

Don't be afraid of the measurements. Just like every great company tracks all its data, so does a person who's in charge of a great body. It's a good opportunity to learn how your body reacts to the changes you're implementing. I love the feeling of trying something new, be it a new eating plan or a new workout routine, for six weeks, and then getting feedback through my measurements to see what changed. When you see those big changes, it's so motivating to either continue the same plan or to change it up and see if you can improve on those numbers again. Have fun with it. After all, life is meant to be fun. Don't take this process too seriously; this shouldn't be a burden or a chore.

Step 3: Discipline

While I encourage you to have fun, it's also important to remember that this process does require a fair amount of Discipline. Although I don't want you to see this as a burden or a chore, creating discipline is going to get uncomfortable at times, particularly in the beginning. Yes, getting up early to work out is never going to become 'fun', but you can make sure the workout itself is enjoyable. I never like getting up early, but I always love it when I finish my morning routine and I can give myself a pat on the back for achieving something important to me within the first thirty minutes of my day.

Dig into the discomfort of discipline. Remind yourself that where there is discipline, there is freedom. The more disciplined you become, the better your habits will be. Eventually, you won't have to put so much energy and effort into your health and fitness, as it will just become part of who you are and your normal routine. I don't think about whether I'm going to work out anymore – I just do it.

Step 4: Nutrition

Once you've nailed the first three steps of the Personal Revolution process, you can tackle the final two steps: Nutrition and Exercise. Remind yourself that these two steps are fundamental for everyone to improve their health and fitness, but how you go about each step is unique to you. In other words, there really is no right way to go about it. The key is to stick to the plan, enjoy it, and, most importantly, achieve your goals.

Do not overthink your nutritional routine. If you make it complicated, you're more likely to give up. With this in mind, follow healthy eating principles and guidelines rather than specific diets and meal plans. Learn and take ownership of your eating habits. Cook some meals, and prep some food. Who cares if you burn the chicken the first time, or even the second? Figure it out.

Step 5: Exercise

This is the fifth and final step in the Personal Revolution process. As with the previous step, there is no 'right' way to work out. On the contrary, I encourage you to try some different workouts. If you haven't worked out before or haven't done any exercise in a while, spend some time trying out different styles of fitness training, different classes, and so on.

Give yourself the opportunity to see if you like anything new or different in the fitness industry. It's always changing and adapting, so you might be surprised. Even the nature of gyms and studios may surprise you. Maybe what you envision a gym or studio to be is vastly different from what it is now. Reach out to a good trainer, book a consultation to discuss your goals, and create a plan.

YOU CAN DO THIS

Don't think you have to take this journey alone. If you need help, get it. Don't continue doing nothing because you don't know what to do. Just work your way through the steps, one by one. I'm sure that whatever you come up with as your strategy – to become the person you aspire to be – will work for you. Sure, you might need to enlist some help here or there along the way to further that journey, but you can do this. Don't sacrifice your health and fitness any longer for your career, or anything else. Those days are over. It's time to take back control.

Remember, it's your life, your potential, and, most importantly, *your* Personal Revolution.

A SMALL REQUEST

Thank you for reading *Your Personal Revolution*.

If you enjoyed it, I'd be grateful if you'd consider leaving an honest review on Amazon. Your feedback is important to me as an author, and reviews help other readers decide whether to read this book, too.

Jay

ACKNOWLEDGEMENTS

Are you meant to start or end an acknowledgement section by thanking your partner? I don't know, but the first person who came to mind that I need to mention is my wife, Lucy. I must thank her for her unconditional love and support throughout this whole process. The challenges of writing and publishing this book were magnified by COVID-19 and a major house renovation, and I couldn't have done it without her. All you need in life is one person to believe in you 100 per cent and you can achieve more than you can possibly imagine. Lucy is that one person for me. 'Thank you. I love you.'

This book wouldn't have even been a thought in my mind, let alone actually written, if it weren't for Mike Reid from Dent. When I first joined KPI (Key Person of Influence Accelerator), I don't think I believed I would have a fully completed book a year later until I had the first draft in my hand. Mike and his KPI systems allowed me to unpack all the information you have read today and get it onto paper. Having him as a friend, business coach and mentor is so valuable, and I appreciate him in all his capacities. 'Cheers, mate!'

No great book gets published without an amazing publishing company. Here is where Scott MacMillan and the team at Grammar Factory stepped in and got this book over the line for me. Scott was not only crucial in keeping me on track with the timeline of publishing, but he also kept me accountable to the entire process from the day the very first word was put to paper. In order to truly GSD (Get Shit Done), you must have someone holding you accountable on a weekly basis. Scott has been that guy for me. I couldn't have done it without him. '#NoFail'

As you've read in this book, having the support and love from friends and family is a big part of successfully achieving a Personal Revolution. It's important for success in all other aspects of your life, not just health and fitness. My mum and dad, Alison and Daniel, Megan, Adam and Hudson have always supported my decisions, whether they agreed with them or not – the sign of a loving and caring family, for which I am eternally grateful. My 'in-law' family, Dave and Lyn, Marc, Lindsey, Grayson and Max, your support and encouragement never goes unnoticed. As the saying goes, 'You can choose your friends but not your family', so I want them to know I don't take our family relationship for granted. 'Love you all.'

I've read that we are all the average of the five people closest to us, so, considering I have more than five amazing friends, I must be doing better than average! In alphabetical order:

Daniel: a high school mate, a travelling partner, my sounding board, a friend for life.

Greg and Abhay: second-best cottage weekend partners ever!

John: I've waited ten years to be able to acknowledge him in return after he released a CD mix and gave me a shoutout.

John and Chris: escape room specialists and former dance floor partners.

Len: an older brother, a client, an inspiration for this book.

Phil: an uncle, turkey dinner chef and fascinating conversationalist.

Rick and Tom: best cottage weekend partners ever!

Shawn: a best man, a friend, a colleague, a confidant; he wears many hats in my life and he wears them well.

Stephen: first Canadian friend, a FIFA night founder, concert and adventure organizer.

Steve and Salwa: life bookers, sleepover pals, cocktail nights and interesting discussions.

Tamara: a fellow dreamer, a phone caller, deep thoughts and tough conversations.

'You're all the best friends I could ask for.'

And finally, I must acknowledge all the clients and bootcamp members I've had the privilege of working with over all these years. All the expertise and knowledge in this book has come from them. They have opened themselves up to me and I have been able to watch, learn and extract the tricks and tips needed to achieve a Personal Revolution. I've seen them succeed, fail, grow, overcome and excel in their health and fitness journeys and through life itself. As much as I'm a crucial part of their lives, they are crucial to mine. Without them I would be nothing, truthfully.

ABOUT THE AUTHOR

Originally from Australia, Jay moved to Toronto in 2008 with nothing more than a backpack. He worked his way up from the bottom of the corporate gym industry, from Head Personal Trainer, to Group Fitness Manager, to Functional Training Program Director where he was brought back to design, implement and run a fitness program for a number of years. In 2010 he started his first personal training business, while owning and running Buns of Steel, one of Toronto's longest surviving boot camps. In 2016 he was selected as Elite Trainer to provide coaching services for international travelling executives for World Trainer's 'Global Elite Trainer Network'.

Jay played rugby league for the Canadian national team in a tournament in the United States. He has competed in Classic Natural Bodybuilding and Natural Physique shows. He gets called upon regularly to participate in fitness and health product beta testing and was hired to be the trainer and voice actor in a running app that is still in development.

Jay now runs a company called PERSONAL REVOLUTION, where he works exclusively with Toronto's top-tier executives from companies like LCBO, CBC, Dyson, Apple and RBC, to name a few. He runs a six-month life transformation program for overworked executives to restore life balance through health and fitness optimization while maintaining their high-functioning careers. A combination of one-on-one coaching, workshops, live events, workouts, and accountability groups creates a unique learning environment and an immersive experience for his clients to experience a Personal Revolution.

CPSIA information can be obtained
at www.ICGtesting.com
Printed in the USA
BVHW032342180621
609394BV00001B/3